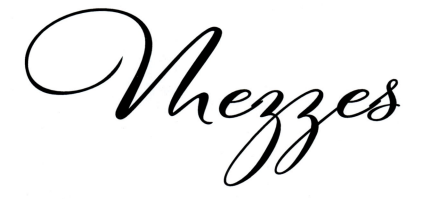

Plant-Based

Salads, Snacks, Dips, Sips, & Sweets

Lisa Sizemore

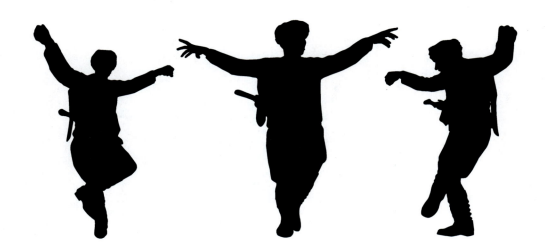

ISBN 979-8-9857238-0-9

Copyright © 2022

Self-Published by Lisa Sizemore, RN HN-BC

Author: Lisa Sizemore Holistic Registered Nurse Board Certified

Front Cover: Baklava with Spiced Almond Syrup & Bitter Dark Chocolate

Book Design, and Photography by Lisa Sizemore

Consultation with Claude Nicholas Arfaras and Dr. April Arfaras

All Rights Reserved - No part of this publication may be reproduced, or stored in a retrieval system, or transmitted in any form or by any means, mechanical, recording or otherwise, without the express written permission of the copyright holder.

Author contact: yiayia2021@gmail.com

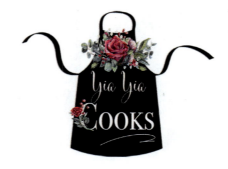

Dedication

Dedicated to my extraordinary family - who just like beloved baklava, is scattered with sweet wonderful nuts.

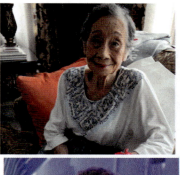
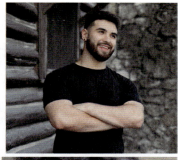
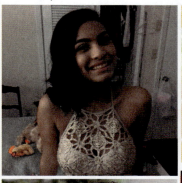
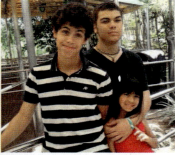
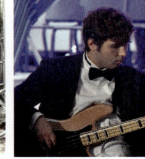
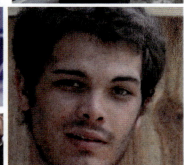
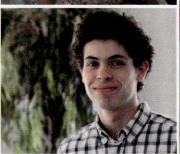
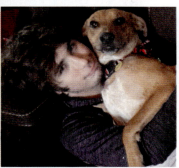
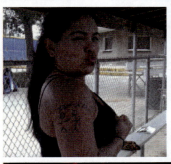
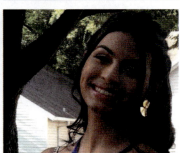
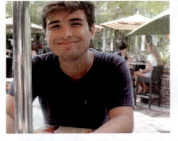
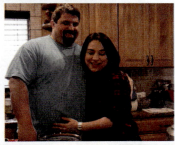
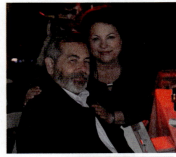
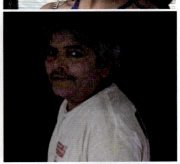
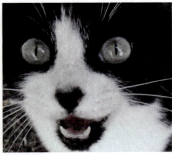
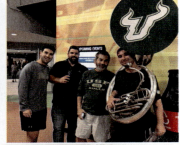
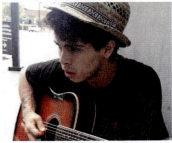
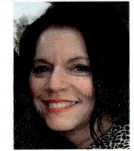
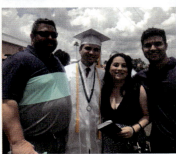
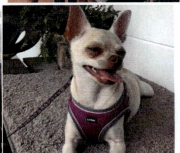
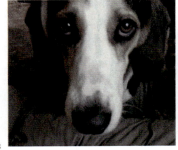
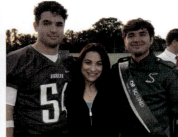

Contents

Dedication	3
Welcome	7
Introduction	8
Definitions	10
Mezze Definition	10
Wholefood Plant-Based Diet Definition	10
Salads	**11**
Greek Salad	12
Greek Potato Salad	13
Massaged Kale Salad with Hummus Dressing	15
Potato Salad with Mint Dressing	16
Chopped Salad with Chickpeas	17
Creamy Cucumber & Tomato Salad with Tzatziki Dressing	19
Greek Village Salad	19
Greek Village Salad with Tzatziki	19
Lentil Salad	21
Fattoush Salad	23
Tabouli with Celery & Mint	25
Holiday Tabouli	25
Tomatoes with Fresh Mint	26
Fruit Salad with Mint & Cinnamon Simple Syrup	27
Orange Slices & Pomegranate Seeds	29
in Spiced Wine Syrup	29
Salad Dressings	**30**
Greek Salad Dressing	31
Greek Hemp Dressing	31
Hummus Salad Dressing	31
Mint Salad Dressing	32
Tahini Dressing	33
Tzatziki Dressing	33
Dips & Smears	**34**
Almond Pate	35
Hummus	35
Plain Hummus	35
Beetroot Hummus	37
Cilantro Hummus	37
How to Roast Beet(s)	37
Greek Roasted Eggplant Spread	39
Roasted Red Bell Pepper	40
Hummus	40
Raw Zucchini Hummus	40
Santorini Yellow Fava	41
Hummus	41
Walnut Spread	43
Noshes & Nibbles	**44**
Baby Beets with Cream Cheese & Pistachios	45
Beer Batter Recipe	47
Beer Battered Blossoms & Veggies	48
Beer Battered "Cardoona"	49
Beer Battered Oysters	51
Greek Oyster Po Boy	51

Tzatziki Tartar Sauce	51
Bruschetta Greek Style	53
Cracked Marinated Olives	54
Olive Tapenade	55
Veggie Fritters	57
Zucchini Fritters	57
Spinach Fritters	57
Tomato Fritters	57
Green Falafels	58
Feta Plate	60
Greek Gazpacho	61
Fried Polenta	63
Greek Guac	65
Fruit Plate	66
Veggie Platter	69
Gyro Slider with Grilled Veggies	70
Grilled Veggie Platter	71
Tempeh Gyro Slider	73
Green Gyro	73
Potato Skins Greek Style with Lemon & Oregano	74
Greek Nachos	75
Keftedes	76
Everyday Koliva	78
Horta - Greens	79
Horta Hand Pie	79
Lemony Greek Roasted Potatoes	80
Persian Pizza	81
Power Greens in Phyllo recipe	83
Tomato Keftedes	84
Stuffed Celery & Other Veggies	85
White Beans on Grilled Greek Toast	86

Quick Pickles 88

Pickled Grapes	89
Pickled Red Onions	89
Pickled Prunes	90
Pickled Carrots	90
Pickled Turnips	91
Sweet Spiced Pickled Figs Stuffed with Feta	93
Pickled Beets	94

Sweets 95

Apple Slices with Agave & Cinnamon	95
Baklava Bon Bons	97
Saragli	97
Chia Pudding with Whiskey Macerated Raisins	99
Cinnamon Nice Cream with Baklava Spiced Nuts	101
Baklava Spiced Nuts	101
Greek Coffee Granita with Cardamom	102
Fig & Anise	103
Energy Bites	103
Fig Granita	105
Dark Chocolate Dipped Figs with Pistachios & Anise Dust	107
Fig Fruit & Nut Salami	108
Fruit with Almond Cream Syrup & Yogurt	109
Medjool Dates with Walnut Stuffing	110
Naked Baklava	111
Naked Fig & Nut Cookie Bites - Skaltsounia	112
Roasted Fruit with Balsamic Cinnamon Syrup	113
Spoon Sweets for a New Day	115
Roasted Pumpkin Spoon Sweet Recipe	117

Loukoumades with Flax Seeds & Greek Coffee Glaze. . . 118

    Greek Coffee Glaze 118

Pita Cinnamon Toast 119

    Cinnamon Sugar 119

Baklava with Spiced Almond Milk Syrup & Bitter Dark Chocolate 121

    Spiced Almond Milk Syrup 121

Sips & Swigs 122

Almond Cream Soda 122

Greek Coffee 123

Greek Whipped Coffee Frappe 124

Horta & Beet Liqueur Shots 125

Iced Orange Tea with 126

Cinnamon & Mint 126

Shepherd's Tea or Mountain Tea 127

Sparkling Mint Punch with Wheatgrass 128

More Yummies 129

Air Fried Almonds with Greek Seasoning. 130

    Oven Roasted Almonds with Greek Seasoning 130

Air Fried Chickpeas with Greek Seasoning 131

    Oven Roasted Chickpeas with Greek Seasoning 131

Almond Coconut Cream 132

Almond Pulp Cookies 133

Almond Cream Syrup 134

Dukkah with Hemp 135

Bread – A Greek Love Affair 136

Greek Kale Chips 139

    Dehydrated Kale Chips 139

    Oven Baked Kale Chips 139

Fig & Raisin Fruit Paste with Anise & Cinnamon 141

Apricot or Date Paste 141

Greek Seasoning Blend 142

Gremolata 142

Grilled Greek Toasts 143

Balsamic Cinnamon Syrup 143

Grilled Pita Breads 143

Mint & Cinnamon Simple Syrup 143

Orange Spiced Wine Syrup 144

Spiced Wine Syrup 144

Wet Walnuts in Spiced Wine Syrup 144

Pita Chips 145

Prosphoro - Greek Offering Bread 146

Schug 148

Zaatar Crackers Recipe 150

Greek-ish Pantry 151

    Greek Spice List 151

    Greek Herbs List 152

    Shopping 153

References 155

Index 157

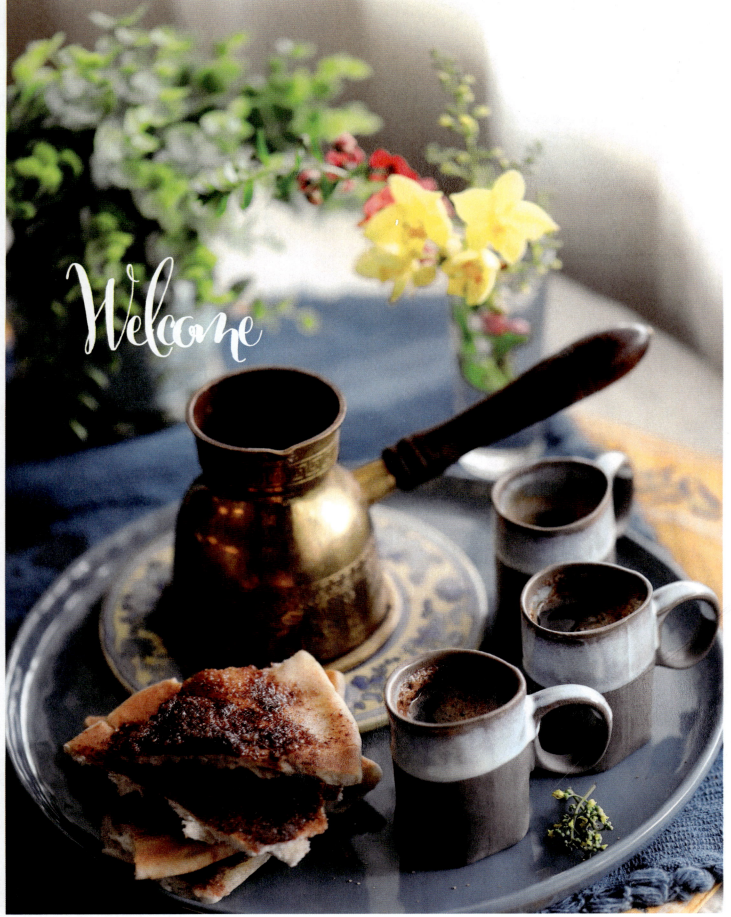

Introduction

Welcome to my Greek American mezze table!

Mezzes are an ancient custom of hospitality. They are a collection of small dishes similar to appetizers or Spanish tapas, but more substantial. The mezze experience is as much about socializing as it is about food. It can be as simple as offering a cookie with coffee or can provide an entire meal - but without an entree. The variety of mezzes is limited only by the cook's imagination. Mezze recipes reflect the season and respect the religious restrictions of the Orthodox community.

In Greek culture, mezze dishes are often served with alcohol, and ouzo is a favorite. Ouzo is a dry distilled anise-flavored aperitif sipped to stimulate the appetite and foster conversation. Greeks love to expound on its many health benefits. I find its flavor to be harsh, so I rarely drink it. My personal choice of beverages are teas, sparkling fruited water, juice shots, and chilled wine.

My love for mezzes began when I was a young child. My father was a Greek immigrant. When he was 10, his family traveled from Greece and settled into a small Greek community here in America. It's where he met and married my Irish mother – and it's the place where we lived until my teens – beloved Tarpon Springs.

Tarpon Springs is located on the west coast of Florida and rests on the Gulf of Mexico. Wikipedia lists it as the largest community of Greek Americans in the United States. Its laid-back locality revolves around family, friends, and no-fuss fabulous foods. Growing up, I looked forward with impatient affection to mezze get-togethers like birthdays, picnics, festivals, religious events, etc.

Now that I'm a yia yia (Greek grandmother), I cherish taking my grandchildren for walks down one of the main streets of Tarpon – Dodecanes Boulevard. I love to share stories of what it was like growing up in this beautiful, quaint community. Just as my father taught me, I teach them to be mindful of the scents of their heritage. To breathe in the salty Gulf breeze and grilled bouquets of oregano and mint that linger in the air around the little cafes and restaurants that line the boulevard. My favorite season is January through March – when the tourists are in town. During these chilly months, the streets are filled with happy visitors. The winter wind circulates the sweet seductive perfumes of orange and lemon blossoms. Add a clear night sky filled with stars, all is well, and life is good.

Dodecanes Blvd. is where the Sponge Docks are located - it is the heartbeat and essence of "Greektown." True to its name, the Sponge Docks are where the sponger's dock their boats. The Anclote River feeds into the Gulf of Mexico and is located on the north side of the street. The Docks are almost always lined with floating vessels – from small fancy sailboats to timeworn sponging crafts. The sponging business and small eateries have provided financial support to the community since the 1880s.

The Sponge Docks are held dear in the hearts of the locals. When a Greek resident departs this life, it's a tradition that the hearse carries the deceased through the Docks' streets for one last visit. The loved one is then transported to Cicada cemetery, where they are laid to rest. After final prayers, incense, and holy water - the funeral procession circles back to the church for a humble meal or mezze reception, aka, a "meal of blessings" to celebrate God's mercy and the life of the one who has not died but lives in the love of Christ. Delicious mezzes are specially prepared with love and prayers to comfort the mourners and help them begin the healing process.

While I have a few sad memories of the Sponge Docks, I mostly remember them as a place of Glendi – a celebration of the Greek community. Several times a year, festivities occur throughout the weekend from the morning deep into the night. Glendi festivals are magical with the exotic sounds of the bouzouki, spirited dancing, smells, and tastes of mouthwatering Greek foods. These gatherings are a uniquely Greek way to embrace life and reconnect with the traditions of our ancestors. My brother communicates with family and friends from our father's birth island, Symi, in the Aegean Sea. They say there is a Glendi gathering on the island every weekend. To be clear, Glendi are not just for Greeks – everyone is welcomed with open arms! If you haven't already, I hope you'll attend a Greek Festival for a lively and delicious Glendi experience.

I grew up in my yia yia's house. This is where my yia yia and mother taught me how to make fabulous Greek foods. Through the years, I built on the lessons I learned in their kitchen. Throughout my adult life, I expanded on my culinary skills by taking classic and contemporary cooking courses.

I'm a registered nurse but took a 2-year leave from my career to live out one of my dreams. My husband Bruce and I opened a 50-seat restaurant. We named it Saint Francis Cafe. Bruce wanted to call it "Buccaneer Party House Sports Bar Paradise" or something like that – but because I was the chef, and with help from Divine intervention, he settled for St. Francis.

We prepared our menu from scratch (mostly vegetarian), and our only charge was a donation. Our cafe was featured on the Today Show on Thanksgiving morning in 1996. It also received national newspaper attention for our unusual concept and delicious menu. We closed the cafe in 1997 when the city invoked eminent domain to use our property for commercial ventures.

I spent most of my professional life working in clinical settings. But for nearly 16 years, I cooked and nursed in a friary - a monastery for Franciscan Friars. Most of the friars were elderly. I wanted to give them my best effort, so I took alternative healthcare courses to supplement their doctor's care. I used my culinary skills to support their health by integrating plant-based foods into their diet. After several weeks of beans, greens, fruits, seeds, and nuts - each friar stated they felt noticeably better. Their doctors also took note of improvements in their health. The Guardian Friar, Fr. John, said that his dental hygienist was impressed by the change in his gum health. When she asked what he was doing differently for such an improvement, he told her –"It's that crazy nurse – she 'may-ka' me eat grass every day!" In addition to their plant-based meals, I placed a small tray of fresh wheatgrass on the top shelf in their fridge. I encouraged the friars to pinch off a knob of grass each day, chew on it till the sweet was gone, then spit out the fibers.

Working in the friary is where my plant-based mission got serious. The blessings and inspirations I received during my years with the friars set my life on a new path. After experiencing the power in plant energy combined with love and prayers, I furthered my studies. I became a Board-Certified Holistic RN and a Certified Professional Plant-Based Chef - aka, Holistic Chef.

My alternative classes and the friars' health motivated me to re-think many of my family's favorite recipes. Many mezzes are already plant-based - but not all. I made adjustments to enrich their green goodness and supercharge them with superfoods while staying true to my Greek culture's flavors and traditions. But you don't have to be vegan or vegetarian to enjoy plant-based mezzes. They are a delicious way to add nutritious nibbles to every diet.

I use all plants in my recipes. Some are whole others are minimally processed – such as "Milkadamia Butter." I occasionally use raw cane sugar, which is not cooked or bleached, so it retains a few healthy minerals. I also shallow fry some of the veggies. Research at the University of Grenada in Spain shows that frying in olive oil actually adds beneficial polyphenols to the food. The scientists theorize that "possibly" frying with oils other than olive oil is what makes frying unhealthy. There are plans for additional analysis and I'll be watching for updates. My holistic nursing studies also teach that delicious foods make our lives happy and whole. I aspire to create recipes that provide healthy nutrition and are pleasurable at the same time. I believe smaller portions of delicious plant-centric recipes satisfy cravings much more than larger amounts of overly processed foods.

I've always had a love and passion for cooking - and I enjoy sharing my skills by teaching classes at local health food stores. Now that I'm retired, I'm more than excited about writing cookbooks. My recipes are an eclectic mix of Greek-Mediterranean and Middle Eastern flavors with American influence. Some are very simple, others take time. But they're all a no-fuss way to express hospitality at casual gatherings.

With this book's writing, a new circumstance surfaced to add to my mezze venues list. We are currently in isolation with extended family due to Covid 19. I prepare vegan mezzes to kitchen-test recipes and for critiquing. I hope the foods at my gatherings will help keep us healthy and create positive energy. Each mezze carries a story. Each gathering provides an opportunity to share those stories and talk about our family's unique history. We come together with four generations at the table and a new awareness of how important it is to add more plants to our diet.

Bruce, aka Papa, is deaf and forgets to wear his hearing aids. He loves to reminisce about the days he ate Jimbo's pork ribs with abandon. Theia Kelly is 96 and can't remember anything - except how much she misses the nickel slot machines at the casino. Rosey, one of our rescued kitties, wants to be a part of the party. She frequently shows up on the table unannounced and Theia Kelly freaks out! Our gatherings aren't as idyllic as I envisioned. More than ever, we need mouthwatering mezzes to help us journey through our new reality.

Time to break out the ouzo - pour me a double, please.

Cheers - kali orexi!

Lisa

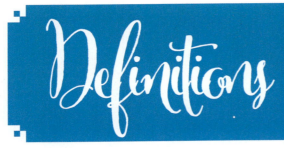

Definitions

Mezze Definition

Delicious foods are central to the joys of life.

Mezzes are more a concept than an established array of dishes. These small plate foods can be eaten as a main course or an appetizer. It all depends on how they're served! They have their roots in Ancient Greece, when drinking establishments were forbidden to serve patrons alcohol unless they were eating something.

Mezzah, Mezzeh

Damascus suburb

Mezze, Mezzes, Mezzedhes

Cyprus and the Balkans

Mazza

Turkey

Mazza

Middle East

Mezzano

Italy – foods "in between" the meal

Mazzot

Hebrew may be related? But includes only unleavened foods

Wholefood Plant-Based Diet Definition

A plant-based diet consists mostly or entirely of foods derived from plants, including vegetables, grains, nuts, seeds, legumes and fruits, and with few or no animal products. A plant based-diet is not necessarily vegetarian. The use of the phrase plant-based has changed over time, and examples can be found of the phrase "plant-based diet" being used to refer to vegan diets, which contain no food from animal sources, to vegetarian diets which may include dairy and/or eggs but no meat, and to diets with varying amounts of animal-based foods, such as semi-vegetarian diets which contain small amounts of meat. (Wikipedia)

My mezze recipes are completely constructed with plants that are mostly minimally processed.

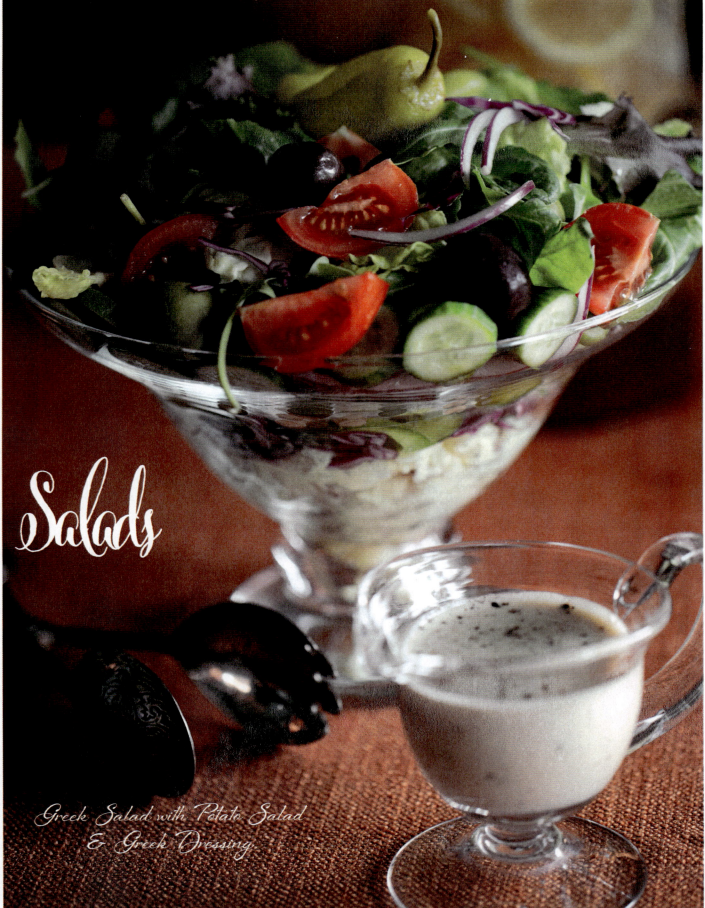

Salads

Greek Salad with Potato Salad & Greek Dressing

Greek Salad

Makes 4 to 8 mezze portions

Our award-winning Greek Salad was the most popular item on the menu at our little restaurant, Saint Francis Cafe. We layered it on top of Greek potato salad or wrapped in a warm pita or naan slathered with homemade hummus.

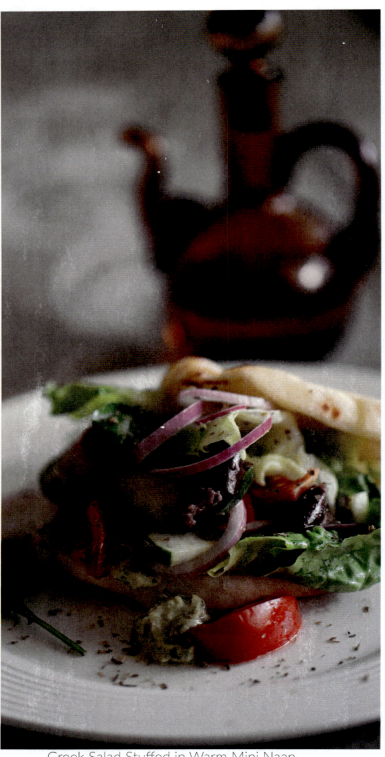

Greek Salad Stuffed in Warm Mini Naan

Ingredients

- 6.5 ounce bag of sweet butter lettuce or your favorite lettuce
- 2 small tomatoes, like Campari variety, sliced
- ¼ red onion sliced or diced
- 2 Persian or mini cucumbers sliced
- 6 each Kalamata and Castelvetrano olives
- 4 to 6 Greek peppers
- 2 ounces plant-based feta cheese like Violife brand
- Pinch of dried oregano
- 1 recipe "Greek Potato Salad" on page 13

Directions

1. Spoon potato salad into bottom of medium salad bowl.
2. Toss veggies separately in a medium bowl with "Greek Salad Dressing" on page 31 then layer veggies onto the potato salad.
3. Cut 1 quarter of the plant feta into small cubes or pinch small pieces off of the slab and place onto the salad.
4. Top with Greek peppers and olives.
5. Sprinkle with pinch of dried oregano.
6. Serve immediately.

Greek Potato Salad

Makes 8 to 12 mezze portions.

Greek Potato Salad is the first mezze to disappear.

Ingredients

- 2 lbs. small or baby potatoes, unpeeled and scrubbed clean
- ½ small sweet onion diced
- 1 small bunch green onions (5), thinly sliced, including green part
- 1 green bell pepper or red bell pepper diced
- ½ cup dill pickles diced

Greek Potato Salad Dressing

- 1 1/4 cups vegan mayonnaise or more to taste
- 1 tablespoon extra-virgin olive oil
- 1-tablespoon apple cider vinegar
- 1 teaspoon dried dill
- ½ teaspoon dried mint
- ½ teaspoon ground oregano
- ½ teaspoon sea salt
- Few grinds of fresh milled pepper

Directions Dressing

1. In a medium bowl whisk together the mayonnaise, olive oil, vinegar, dill, mint, oregano, sea salt, and pepper -
2. Proceed with recipe as directed.

Directions Potato Salad

1. Potato salad is best if made while potatoes are still warm so they absorb the dressing.
2. Add the potatoes to the dressing mixture and toss to coat. They may break apart a little, this adds to the creaminess of the salad.
3. Add the green onions, sweet onion, bell pepper, and dill pickles.
4. Toss all ingredients together.
5. Serve immediately or chilled.
6. Store covered in the refrigerator for up to 3 days

Potato Cooking Directions

1. Scrub potatoes and leave peels on.
2. Place whole potatoes in large pot, cover with cool water, and bring to a boil over medium high heat.
3. Reduce heat to simmer and cook approximately 20 to 25 minutes or until the potatoes are tender when pierced with a knife.
4. Drain well after cooking – when cool enough to handle, cut each potato into quarters and proceed with potato salad recipe.

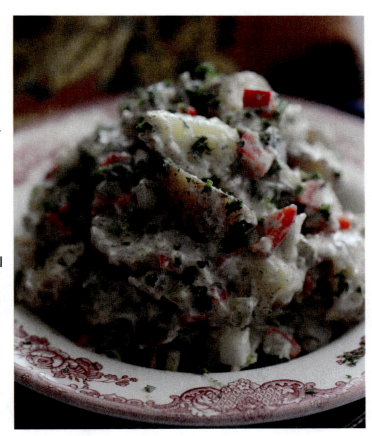

Greek Potato Salad

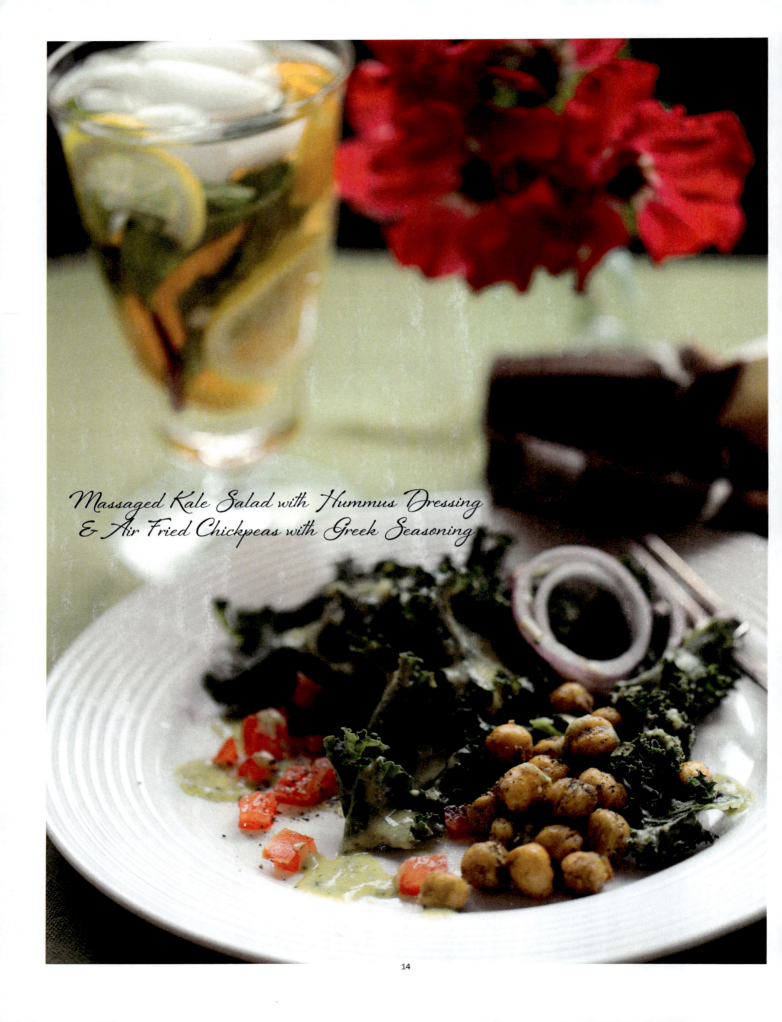

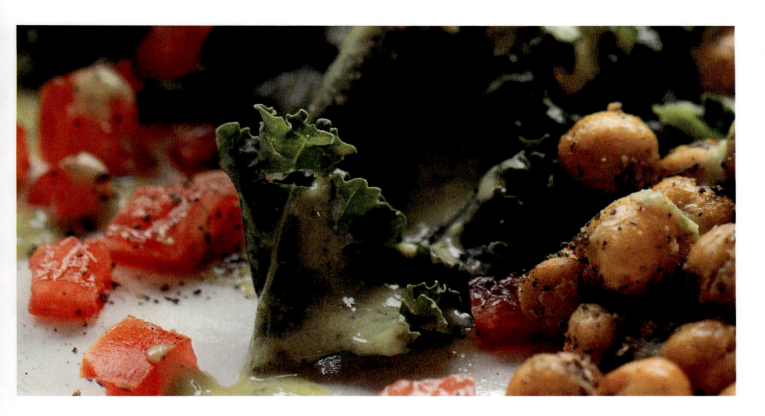

Massaged Kale Salad with Hummus Dressing

Makes 6 to 8 mezze servings

Kale is an antioxidant-rich, superfood superstar. I often add it to our meals and green juice shots. It also makes a mouth-watering Greek salad — but curly leaf kale can be very tough. Raw food cooking classes taught me how to massage the leaves to make them luscious and tender. I remember being so impressed that I couldn't wait to make massaged kale salads for my family and for the friars. I also love to share kale salads at work and picnics.

Life is busy and many people don't cook because they are exhausted and cooking can be time consuming and burdensome. However, preparing meals at home is vital for nurturing good health, and it can be enjoyable and easy. One taste of an incredible salad may just be the light that inspires the birth of a plant-based foodie.

Ingredients

- 1 bunch curly kale
- 2 Roma tomatoes, remove seeds, dice into small cubes
- ¼ red onion sliced into rings
- "Hummus Salad Dressing" on page 31
- Optional: 1 cup "Air Fried Chickpeas with Greek Seasoning" on page 131or plain canned chickpeas.

Directions

1. Wash kale thoroughly.
2. Remove stems, tear kale leaves into bite-size pieces.
3. Add kale leaves to large bowl and add a tablespoon of hummus dressing.
4. Toss and scrunch the kale with your hands to soften the leaves.
5. Add diced tomatoes, sliced red onion, and hummus dressing.
6. Toss to coat the veggies in the dressing.
7. Add a little unrefined sea salt and pepper if desired.
8. Serve chilled.

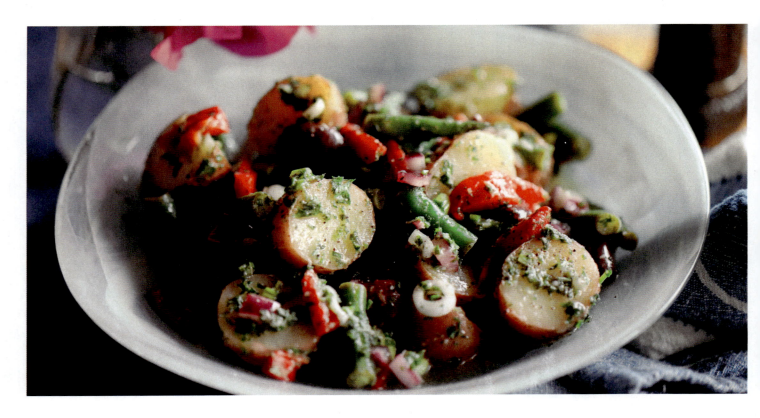

Potato Salad with Mint Dressing

Makes 4 to 6 mezze portions.

Ingredients
- 1 pound small potatoes scrubbed clean
- 1 cup of fresh green beans, blanched and cut into ½ inch pieces
- 1 roasted red bell pepper from a jar, drained, and cut into strips
- ½ red onion coarsely chopped
- 8 Kalamata or Greek black olives, cut into halves
- 1 small bunch of curly parsley leaves, finely chopped
- 1 recipe "Mint Salad Dressing" on page 32
- Unrefined sea salt and freshly milled black pepper to taste

Directions
1. Place whole potatoes in medium saucepan and cover with cool water.
2. Bring to a boil on high heat – reduce heat to a simmer and simmer for 15 to 20 minutes or until fork tender.
3. Drain the potatoes in a colander and cool until able to handle.
4. For the green beans – fill a small pot with water, add a teaspoon of salt, and bring to a boil over high heat.
5. Add the green beans and boil until the beans turn bright green – 1 to 2 minutes.
6. Drain the beans and transfer to a bowl filled with ice and water.
7. Once the beans are room temperature, drain, and cut into 1/2 -inch pieces.
8. Cut potatoes into halves and place in a medium bowl.
9. Toss the potatoes with the green beans, red bell pepper strips, onion slices, olives, parsley, and the mint dressing.
10. Sprinkle with unrefined sea salt to desired taste, and a few grinds of freshly milled pepper.
11. Toss with finely chopped curly parsley.
12. This potato salad is best if served slightly warm or at room temperature shortly after it's made. But it will keep for 3 days, covered in the refrigerator – but the flavors and colors fade.

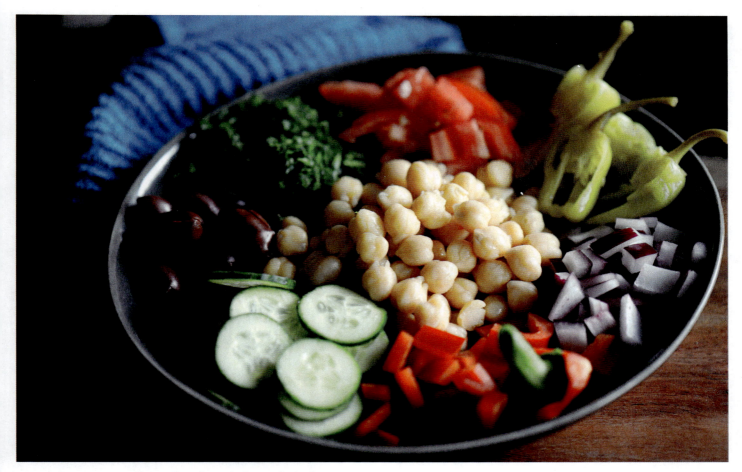

Chopped Salad with Chickpeas

Makes 4 to 6 mezze portions.

Ingredients

- 15 ounce can chickpeas drained and rinsed
- 2 Roma tomatoes diced
- ¼ red onion diced
- 2 Persian or mini cucumbers sliced
- 1 small bunch curly parsley finely chopped
- 6 Kalamata olives chopped
- 2 to 3 Greek peppers cut into halves lengthwise
- 1 recipe "Mint Salad Dressing" on page 32 or other dressing of choice

Directions

1. Mix beans and veggies together.
2. Toss with dressing.
3. Serve immediately or chilled.

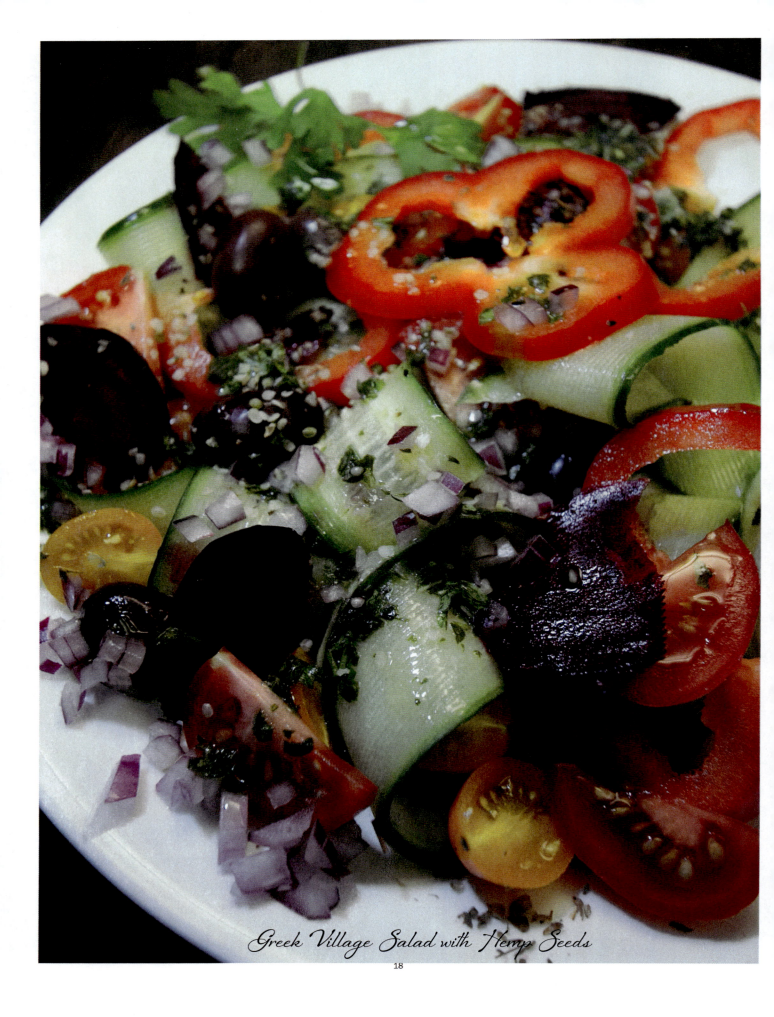
Greek Village Salad with Hemp Seeds

Creamy Cucumber & Tomato Salad with Tzatziki Dressing

Makes 4 to 6 mezze servings.

Ingredients

- 1 English or hothouse cucumber sliced into rounds
- 6 grape tomatoes cut into halves
- ¼ red onion cut into thin slices
- 1/3 cup "Tzatziki Dressing" on page 33
- Unrefined sea salt and freshly milled pepper to taste

Directions

1. Toss all ingredients together in a medium bowl.
2. Add salt and pepper to taste.
3. Serve chilled.
4. Store covered in refrigerator for 2 to 3 days.

Greek Village Salad

Makes 4 to 6 mezze servings.

Ingredients

- 1 green bell pepper cut into bite sized pieces
- 1 orange or red bell pepper cut into bite sized pieces
- 1 small purple onion cut into thin slices or diced
- 1 hothouse cucumber sliced into rounds - or thinly sliced into strips w veggie peeler
- 1 small roasted beet thinly sliced w veggie peeler.
- 12 grape tomatoes cut into quarters
- 1 recipe "Greek Salad Dressing" on page 31
- Thin slice of vegan feta for each serving
- 2 teaspoons capers drained
- Greek pepperoncini for each serving
- Pinch of dried oregano
- Optional thin slices of beets and hemp seeds

Directions

1. Place green & orange bell peppers, onion slices, cucumbers and grape tomatoes into medium sized bowl.
2. Toss with Greek Salad Dressing to coat veggies.
3. Place pieces of vegan feta on top of veggies.
4. Top salad with capers, pepperoncini, sprinkle with oregano & optional hemp seeds.
5. Serve immediately.

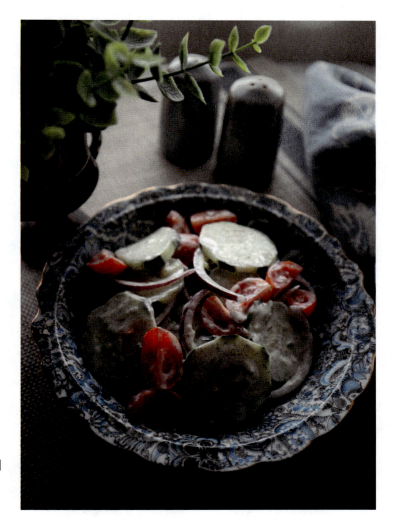

Greek Village Salad with Tzatziki

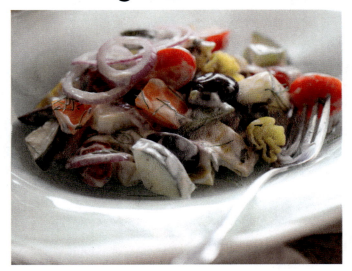

1. Make Greek Village Salad but omit Greek Salad Dressing and toss with 1/2 cup of Tzatziki.

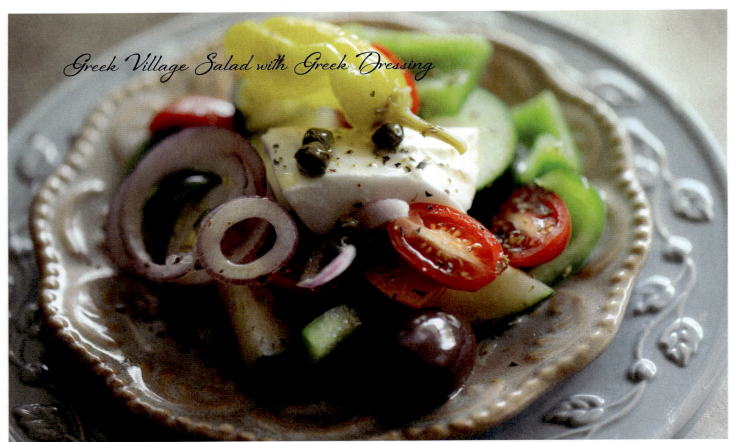
Greek Village Salad with Greek Dressing

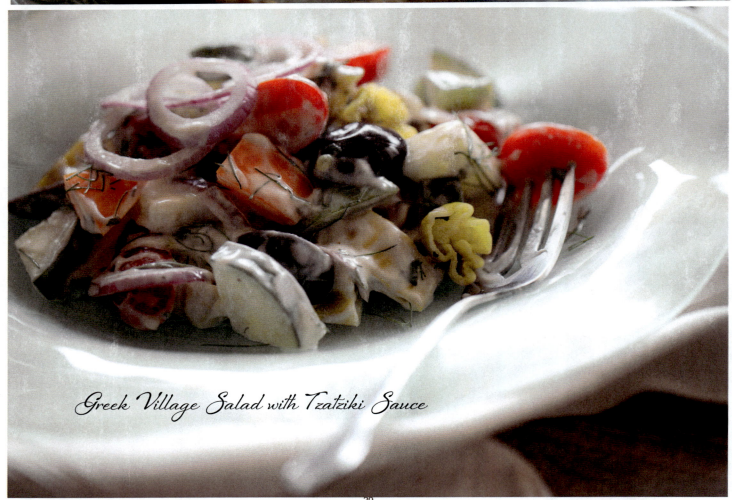
Greek Village Salad with Tzatziki Sauce

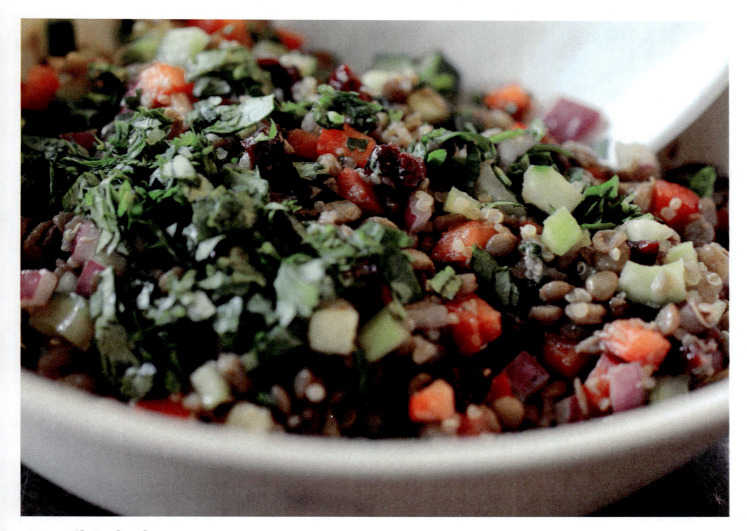

Lentil Salad

Makes 6 to 12 mezze portions

This lentil salad makes detoxing delicious!!!

Ingredients

- 2-1/2 cups cooked lentils
- 1/2 cup red quinoa, cooked
- 2 celery ribs diced
- 1 red bell pepper diced
- 2 mini cucumbers diced
- 1/2 red onion diced
- 3/4 cup dried cranberries
- 1-tablespoon extra-virgin olive oil
- 2 tablespoons raw vinegar with mother
- 1-tablespoon fresh lime juice
- 1-teaspoon lime zest from organic lime
- 2 tablespoons Nama Shoyu (raw, unpasteurized soy sauce) or Braggs Aminos
- 1-teaspoon maple syrup or agave
- 1 bunch cilantro chopped

Directions

1. Toss all ingredients together.
2. Serve chilled.

Note:

The special ingredient that sets this salad apart and makes this salad so delicious is Nama Shoyu, or raw soy sauce. I learned about this sauce at my raw cooking and macrobiotic classes. It's a little pricey but worth every penny.

This recipe makes a good amount of delicious Lentil Salad. In addition to your mezze table, consider sharing it at a picnic or workplace potluck.

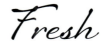

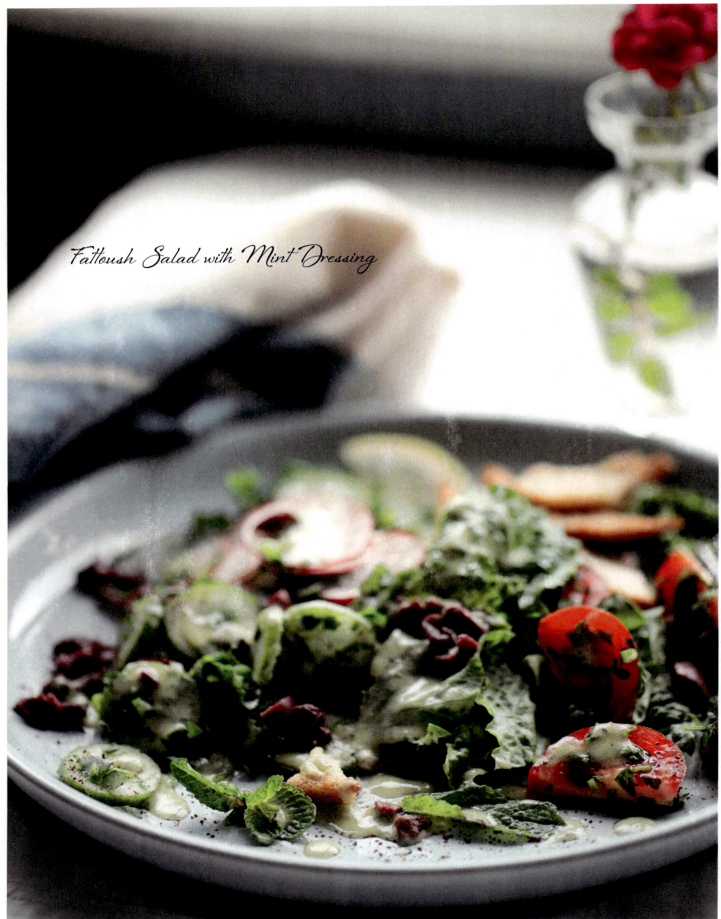
Fattoush Salad with Mint Dressing

Fattoush Salad

Makes 4 to 8 servings.

Pass the napkins, because Fattoush is most definitely a drool-luscious salad.

Fattoush is a mouthwatering Middle Eastern salad that's lemony and delish! My first fattoush experience was at a local Persian restaurant, and it was YUM at first bite! So I just had to share a recipe for fattoush in my cookbook.

It's similar to tabouli, but there's no parsley and the veggies are cut into larger pieces. Instead of using bulgur wheat, fattoush is made with air dried or toasted pita pieces, flatbread, or naan. In addition to fresh lemon juice, the salad is traditionally sprinkled with sumac, enhancing its tart lemony flavor.

My version is especially yummy because it's made with creamy Hummus Dressing with Cilantro (see recipe for Hummus Salad Dressing). Plus, I toss in a little Romaine lettuce and chopped Kalamata olives to Greek-a-fy it.

Ingredients

- 1 pita, flatbread or naan, cut or torn into bite-sized pieces
- Drizzle bread pieces with olive oil, a light sprinkle of salt, and bake on the center rack on a parchment lined baking sheet in a 350°F preheated oven for 10 to 15 minutes or until golden – turn halfway through baking.
- 2 Roma or Campari tomatoes sliced
- 2 Persian or mini cucumbers sliced
- ½ sweet onion sliced
- 4 radishes thinly sliced
- 1 bunch curly parsley finely chopped
- Leaves from 6 stems of mint
- 1 small head of Romaine lettuce torn into bite-sized pieces
- 8 Kalamata olives chopped
- 1 recipe "Hummus Salad Dressing" on page 31
- 2 teaspoons sumac

Directions

1. Toast pieces of bread as directed and cool to room temperature – maybe toasted a day ahead, cooled, and stored in Ziploc bag or another sealed container.
2. In a medium bowl mix the tomatoes, cucumbers, onion, radishes, parsley, mint, and olives together.
3. Toss salad with Hummus Dressing
4. Top with toasted pieces of pita and sprinkle with sumac.
5. Serve immediately.

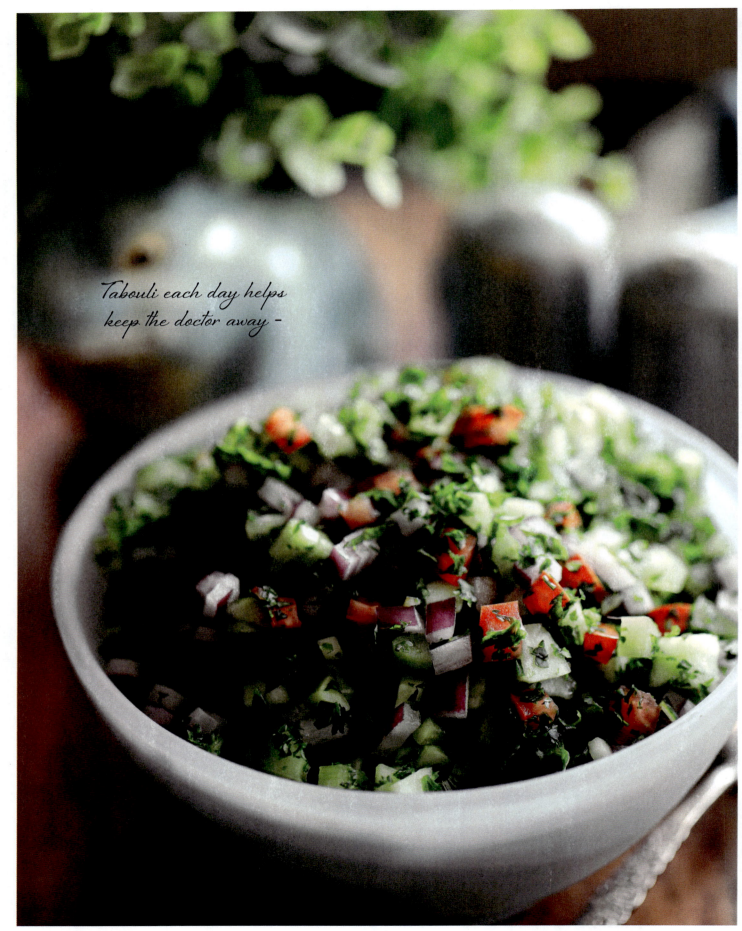

Tabouli each day helps keep the doctor away –

Tabouli with Celery & Mint

Makes 4 to 6 mezze portions

Tabouli is a Mediterranean salad. Its main ingredients are parsley, mint, and cracked wheat. For this recipe, I replaced the wheat with celery. It makes a delicious mezze, and a detox powerhouse.

From a very young age, my father encouraged my siblings and me to eat parsley. We grew up eating (mostly protesting) the curly variety. As an adult, I came to love and appreciate the healthy gift of parsley. I almost always have a bunch on hand. I use a lot of Italian parsley, but curly parsley holds up best in cold salads like tabouli.

I regularly put together a tabouli for my mezze gatherings. It's simple to prepare; it adds flavor and makes a beautiful appetizer. Plus, it's packed with nutrients. I serve it as a salad or on hummus, veggie burgers, and falafel wraps. Leftovers can be used as a garnish for soup.

Ingredients
- 3 celery finely diced
- 1 small bunch curly parsley finely chopped (curly holds up better than Italian parsley)
- 1 small bunch fresh mint leaves finely chopped
- 2 Persian or mini cucumbers finely diced
- 2 Roma tomatoes finely diced
- ¼ red onion finely diced
- 1 garlic clove finely minced or mashed
- 2 tablespoons fresh lemon juice
- 2 tablespoons olive oil
- ½ teaspoon unrefined sea salt
- Optional: 1 tablespoon hemp seed hearts

Directions
1. Toss all ingredients together.
2. Serve chilled.
3. I prefer to serve tabouli on the same day it's made. It will keep in the refrigerator for 2 to 3 days but the green color of the parsley and mint sometimes fades.
4. Optional: add a tablespoon of hemp hearts.

Holiday Tabouli

Make Tabouli recipe, but omit the garlic and tomatoes. Add seeds from 1 pomegranate, ½ cup dried cranberries, 2 teaspoons maple syrup (or more to your taste), and a pinch of ground cinnamon.

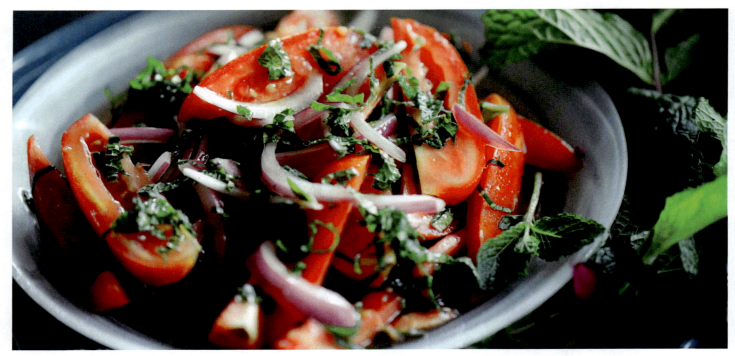

Tomatoes with Fresh Mint

Makes 4 to 6 mezze portions.

"A world without tomatoes is like a string quartet without violins."

Laurie Colwin

My family has a deep affection for tomatoes. Growing up, we ate them in one form or another almost every day. My parents refused to buy them from the grocery store. They insisted on driving to country stands that sold tomatoes fresh from the vine. Each summer, my mother would purchase them by the bushel and can them. This way, we would have tomatoes through the fall and winter months.

Mint grew wild all over Tarpon Springs and was commonly used by the Greek cooks in the community. It flourished in my yia yia's side yard and was one of her favorite herbs. I love the way mint gives my tomato salad a fresh taste of the Mediterranean and mouthwatering memories of my yia yia's kitchen.

Ingredients

- 3 plum tomatoes, cut each into 8ths
- ¼ red onion cut into thin slices
- 16 fresh mint leaves cut into thin strips
- 1 tablespoon fresh lemon juice
- 1 teaspoon apple cider vinegar
- 2 tablespoons olive oil
- ¼ teaspoon unrefined sea salt

Directions

1. Wash tomatoes thoroughly with cool water.
2. Cut each tomato in half lengthwise – then cut each half into 4 slices – place in small bowl.
3. Cut ¼ piece of red onion into thin slices, and add to tomatoes.
4. Stack mint leaves on top of each other, roll, and slice the roll into thin strips (this is a chiffonade cut), sprinkle onto tomatoes and onions.
5. Add the lemon juice, vinegar, olive oil, and sea salt – toss until the veggies and mint are coated.
6. Serve chilled or at room temperature.
7. Best if served on the same day – the lemon juice causes the mint to lose its fresh green color after 3-4 hours. But the salad is still yummy the next day.

If there are any leftover tomatoes, they make a slurpy, delicious sandwich on Greek bread, slathered with plant-based mayo – but always alone and over the kitchen sink.

Fruit Salad with Mint & Cinnamon Simple Syrup

Makes 4 to 6 mezze portions.

Ingredients

- Seeds from 1 pomegranate
- 1 seedless orange cut into segments
- 1 kiwi sliced into 8 wedges
- 1/2 cup grapes sliced into halves
- 1 cup strawberries sliced
- 1 Recipe "Mint & Cinnamon Simple Syrup" on page 143
- A few fresh mint leaves & thin lemon slices for garnish

Directions

1. In medium bowl, toss fruit with chilled Mint & Cinnamon Simple Syrup.
2. Serve chilled.
3. Garnish with fresh mint and thin lemon slices.

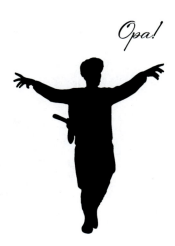

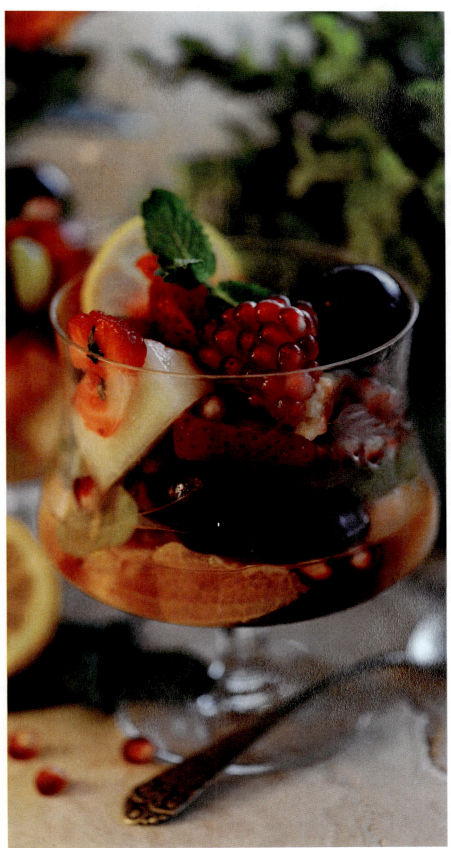

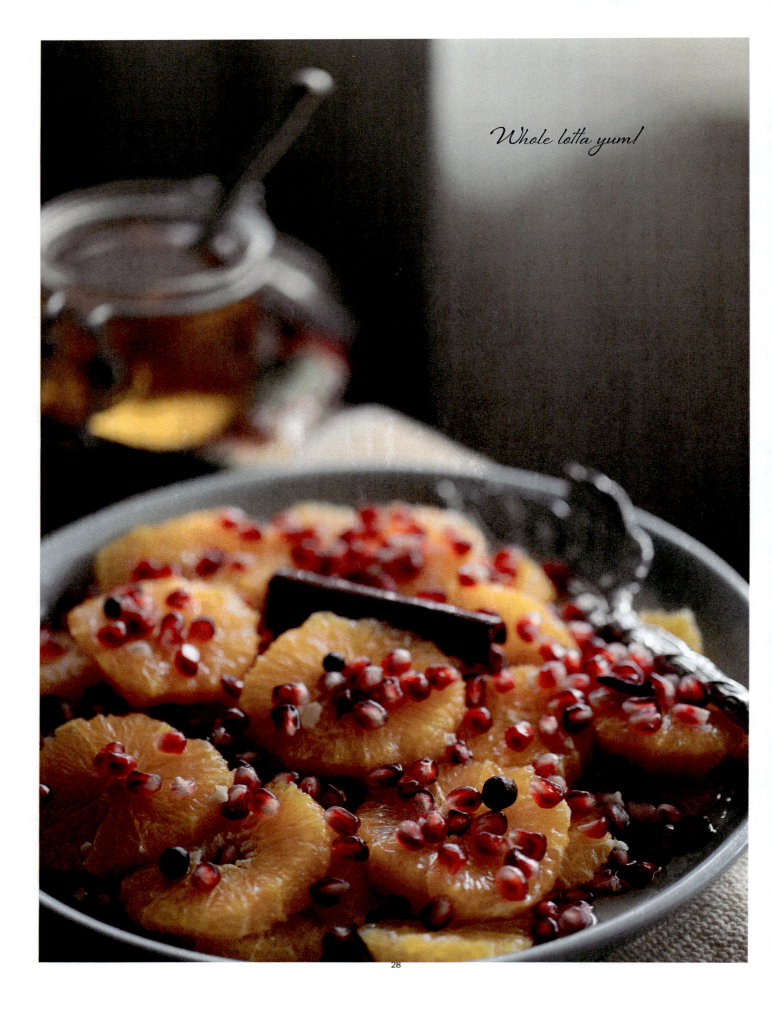

Whole lotta yum!

Orange Slices & Pomegranate Seeds in Spiced Wine Syrup

Makes 24 mezze servings

This recipe was born during a Greek dance for 350 people that I catered at the parish when I worked for Franciscan Friars. The event was so popular we sold out several weeks before the affair. Because of fire ordinance restrictions, we had to turn away many more unhappy patrons at the door.

The day before the dance, I made a tremendous amount of baklava. I ended up with a large amount of leftover soaking syrup and I didn't want the syrup to go to waste. At home, I had 2 orange trees heavy with ripe fruit. I thought oranges macerated in the remaining syrup might make a fabulous dessert or a side – and I was right! Guests couldn't get enough and kept coming back for more.

I've pretty much retired from catering large events. But my niece Lauren was recently married, and I helped out by supplementing her menu with gifts of mezzes. Because my oranges in spiced syrup were so delicious, easy, and beautiful – I added them to the menu. Once again, they were a hit! They were the first mezze to go, not because of the quantity but because those who tried them - came back for 2nds, 3rds, and...

Most of the guests were not aware it was me who made the mezzes. I loved standing near the table and listening to their comments. The oohs and ahs on the deliciousness of the oranges and other mezzes made me smile. The wedding planner asked if I would cater for her company. She said that her accounts included local celebrities and politicians. The minister told me he had performed over 400 weddings with receptions and that my mezzes were "Hands down the most delicious and impressive" he'd ever had. He also asked if I would be interested in providing mezzes for his parishioners' weddings. I explained to both of them that I was enjoying retirement and only made the mezzes as a present for my niece - but I would be happy to send recipes. They were amazed to learn that every mezze – the hummus, the salads, the sauces, and dips were all plant-based.

Ingredients

- 12 oranges peeled and sliced into ¼ to ½ inches
- Seeds from 1 pomegranate (*see note)
- Spiced Wine Syrup
- Ingredients
- 1-cup cane sugar
- 1 cup white wine like Chardonnay
- Rind of ½ organic lemon
- 1 cinnamon stick
- 4 whole cloves
- 4 whole allspice berries
- 1-teaspoon fresh lemon juice

Directions

1. Combine sugar, wine, rind, cinnamon stick, cloves, all allspice in small saucepan
2. Bring to boil over medium high heat - reduce heat and gently simmer syrup for 15 minutes
3. Remove from heat, and cool with spices
4. Once cool, remove spices and lemon rind
5. Stir in fresh teaspoon of lemon juice
6. Spoon cooled syrup onto oranges and pomegranate seeds.
7. Serve chilled.
8. Oranges will keep refrigerated for 1 week.

*Note: Saveur Magazine has instructions on how to easily remove seeds from a pomegranate on YouTube.

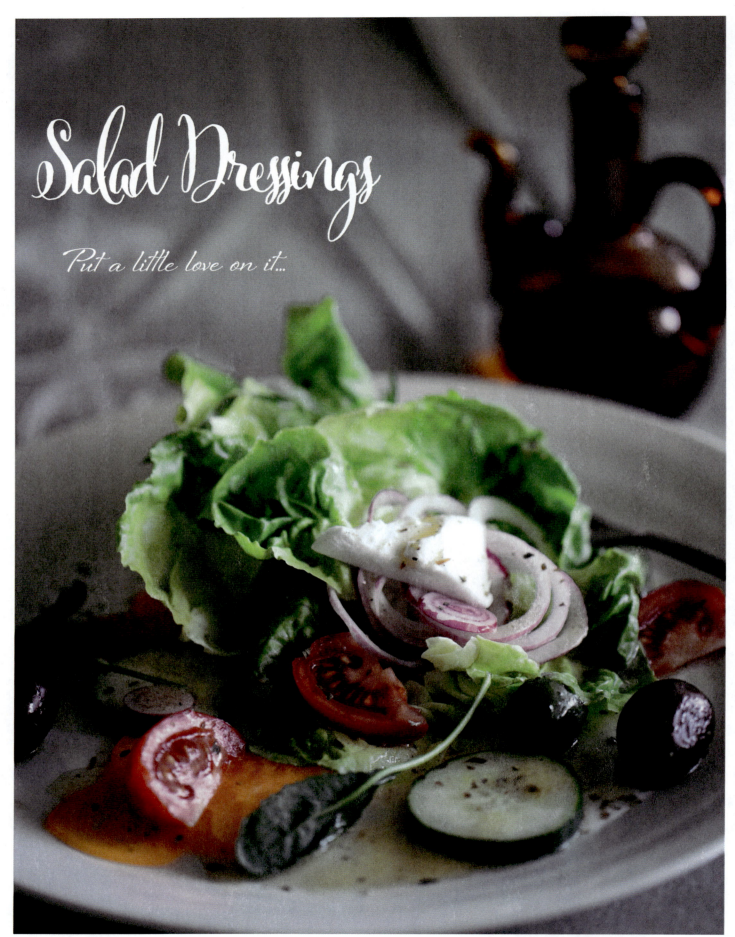

Salad Dressings

Put a little love on it...

Greek Salad Dressing

Ingredients
- ¼ cup olive oil
- 1-tablespoon vinegar
- 2 teaspoons fresh lemon juice
- 1-tablespoon vegan mayonnaise
- 1 teaspoon "Greek Seasoning Blend" on page 142
- OR Instead of Greek Seasoning Blend use 1/4 teaspoon ground dried oregano and 1/2 teaspoon dried mint-
- ¾ teaspoon sea salt or as desired to your taste

Directions
1. Whisk all ingredients together in a small bowl.
2. Store covered in refrigerator.
3. Will keep for up to a week.

Greek Hemp Dressing

Ingredients
- ½ cup hemp seeds soaked 4 hours in water
- 1 mini cucumber (Persian cucumber)
- 2 green onions/scallions including green parts, sliced
- 2 tablespoons apple cider vinegar with mother, like Bragg's brand
- 1-tablespoon fresh lemon juice
- 2-tablespoon extra-virgin olive oil
- 6 fresh mint leaves
- ¼ teaspoon peppercorns
- ½ teaspoon dried ground oregano
- ¾ teaspoon unrefined sea salt

Directions
1. Soak hemp seeds at least 4 hours so dressing will be creamy.
2. Drain hemp seeds.
3. Blitz all ingredients together in blender until lusciously smooth
4. Serve chilled with Tomato Keftedes, on a salad or as a dip for veggies.

Hummus Salad Dressing

Ingredients
- ½ cup "Plain Hummus" on page 35 or your favorite hummus
- 2 tablespoons olive oil
- 2 tablespoons vinegar
- 1-tablespoon fresh lemon juice
- Warm water a teaspoon at a time to thin to your desired thickness

Directions
1. Whisk all ingredients together
2. Toss dressing with salad veggies
3. Serve immediately

Note:

If desired, add an optional 1/4 cup of finely chopped cilantro or mint.

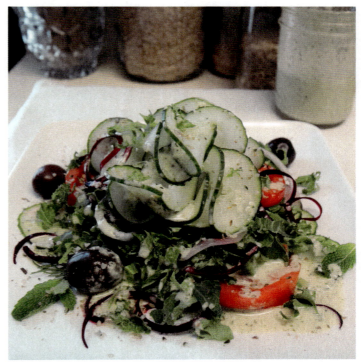

Greek Salad with Hemp Dressing

Nothing dresses up veggies more than an intensely delicious homemade dressing. Flavorful dressings can even entice you to add more health-giving plants to your diet.

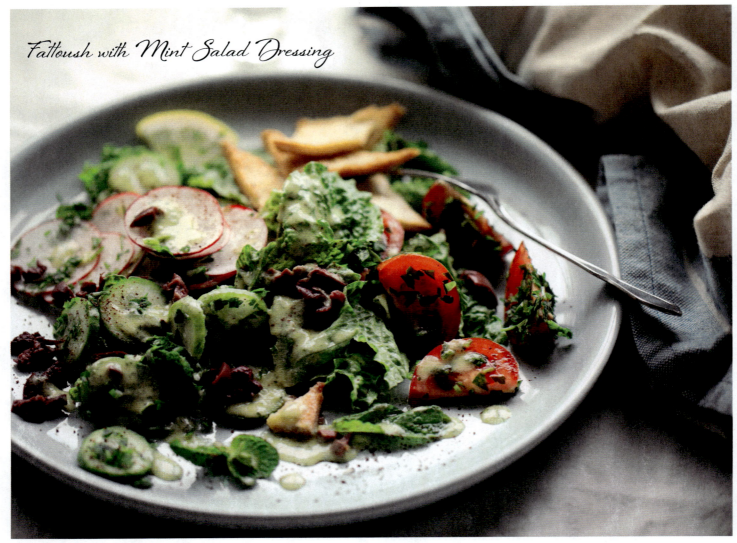
Fattoush with Mint Salad Dressing

Mint Salad Dressing

The perfect dressing is essential to the perfect salad, and I see no reason whatsoever for using a bottled dressing, which may have been sitting on the grocery shelf for weeks, even months - even years.

Julia Child

Delicious on salad, tabouli, or drizzled on veggies.

Ingredients

- 1 garlic clove
- 1/3 cup olive oil
- 1 tablespoon plant-based mayo
- 1 tablespoon fresh lemon juice
- 2 teaspoons apple cider vinegar
- ½ teaspoon unrefined sea salt
- Leaves from 8 sprigs of fresh mint
- Freshly ground black pepper to your desired taste.

Directions

1. Drop garlic clove into blender with motor running to mince.
2. Add olive oil, mayo, vinegar, lemon juice, and salt to blender - blitz until blended and creamy.
3. Add mint – pulse until green specs appear and dressing is smooth.
4. Stir in freshly ground pepper.
5. Transfer to a glass jar with lid.
6. Store in refrigerator for 3 days.

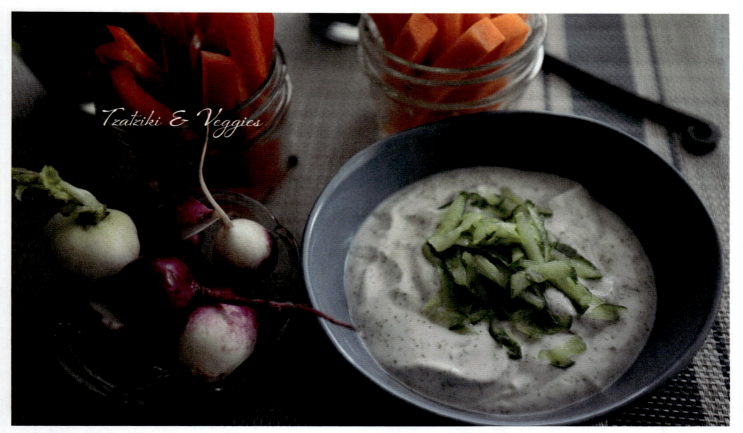

Tahini Dressing

Every brand of tahini I've tried comes separated. There's always a layer of sesame oil at the top of the jar. So I take a moment to stir and blend the tahini before making the dressing.

Ingredients

- 1 garlic clove finely minced
- ½ cup tahini
- ¼ cup lukewarm water or more for a thinner consistency
- 2 tablespoons fresh lemon juice
- ½ teaspoon unrefined sea salt

Directions

1. I use a small food processor to make this dressing and it comes out deliciously creamy.
2. Add minced garlic, tahini, water, lemon juice, sea salt and optional olive oil to bowl of food processor
3. Blitz ingredients until smooth and creamy – scraping the sides of the processor with a spatula as needed
4. Add more water a teaspoon at a time until you reach your desired consistency.

Tzatziki Dressing

Ingredients

- 2 small Persian cucumbers grated with peel
- ½ cup plant based sour cream
- ½ cup plant based mayo - I like Vegenasie
- 2 garlic cloves finely minced
- 1 teaspoon fresh lemon juice
- 2 ½ teaspoons dried dill
- ¼ teaspoon unrefined sea salt
- Optional: fresh dill and mint leaves

Directions

1. Grate cucumbers – gently press between paper towels to absorb excess liquid.
2. In medium bowl whisk together the sour cream, mayo, garlic, lemon juice, dill, cucumbers, and salt.
3. Garnish with optional fresh mint, fresh dill, and /or grated Persian cucumber.
4. Serve chilled.
5. Store in air tight container in fridge.
6. Will keep for 3 to 4 days.

Dips & Smears
Spread the love...

Almond Pate

Almond Pate

Makes 6 to 12 mezze portions.

Ingredients

- 2 cups almonds soaked for at least 4 hours or overnight
- 1 clove garlic, finely minced
- 2 tablespoons fresh lemon juice
- ½ teaspoon unrefined sea salt
- ½ teaspoon ground oregano
- 1 teaspoon Nama Shoyu or Braggs Aminos
- ¼ cup water or more for desired consistency
- 1 tablespoon olive oil or a little more if desired
- ½ red bell pepper finely chopped
- 6 Kalamata olives finely chopped

Directions

1. Drain and rinse almonds.
2. Place almonds in food processor bowl with garlic, lemon juice, salt, ground oregano, shoyu, water, and olive oil.
3. Pulse until fine but not pureed into a butter.
4. Add red bell pepper and olives – finish with a few quick pulses just to mix.
5. Server with crackers, pita chips or as a dip for veggies.
6. Store in refrigerator in air tight container - will keep up to 4 days.

Hummus

No food can get my family (and me) more excited about eating plants than the ancient snack - hummus. I'm totally obsessed with this supreme bean spread. I even imagine Jesus and the Apostles sitting under an olive tree breaking pita to scoop up this creamy, beany goodness from a common bowl.

Hummus is filled with plant protein, is inexpensive, and simple to make. Add a little love energy into the mix, and it's a perfect food! Plus, plain hummus keeps fresh in the fridge for up to a week.

To prevent the transgression of double-dipping, I serve my hummus in a bowl with a spoon. This allows each person to serve up a generous dollop onto their individual plates. Or, you could offer it in small, single-serve bowls.

Plain Hummus

Ingredients

- 1-garlic clove
- 15-ounce can garbanzo beans drained reserve liquid
- 3 tablespoons tahini
- 3 tablespoons olive oil
- 2 tablespoons fresh lemon juice
- 2 tablespoons bean water from can
- ½ teaspoon sea salt
- Pinch ground cumin

Directions

1. With blender running, drop in a garlic clove to mince
2. Add the remaining ingredients: beans, tahini, olive oil, lemon juice, bean water, salt and cumin.
3. Blitz until blended and creamy - add more bean water for desired consistency.
4. Serve at room temperature as a dip for veggies, with "Pita Chips" on page 145.
5. Store in air tight container in refrigerator - will keep up to a week.

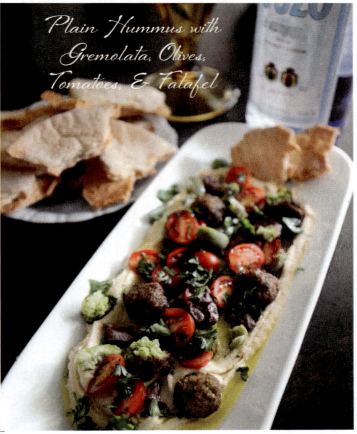

Plain Hummus with Gremolata, Olives, Tomatoes, & Falafel

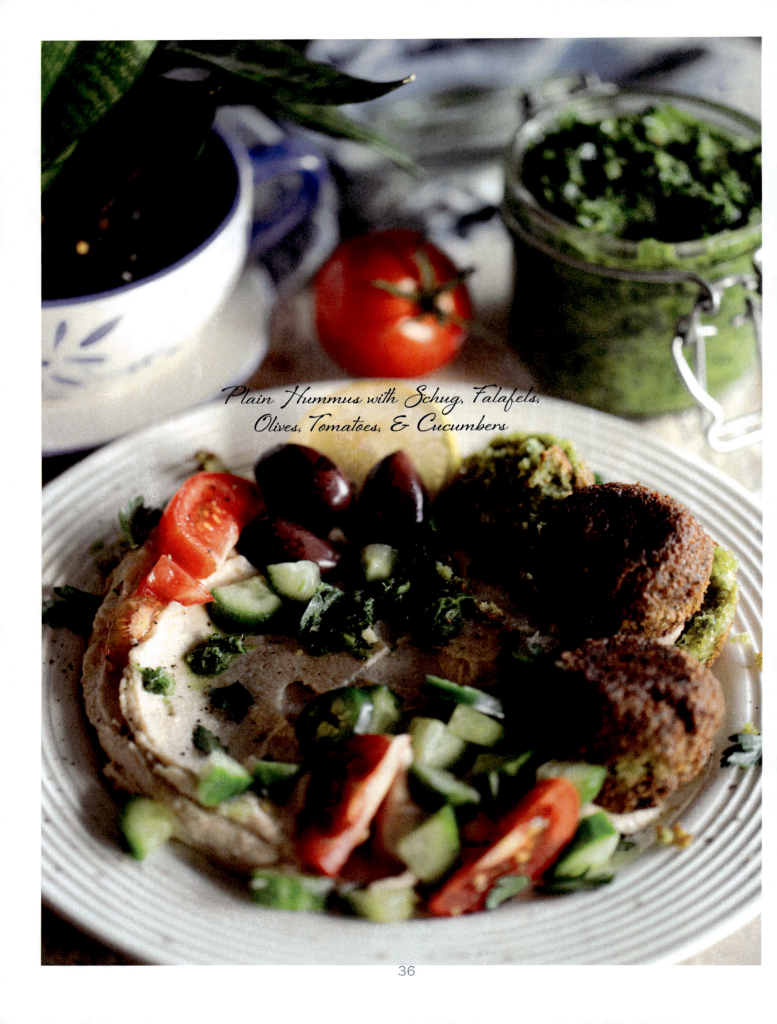

Plain Hummus with Schug, Falafels, Olives, Tomatoes, & Cucumbers

Beetroot Hummus

Ingredients
- 1-garlic clove
- 15-ounce can garbanzo beans drained - reserve bean water
- 1 medium beet, roasted
- 2 tablespoons tahini
- 2 tablespoons fresh lemon juice
- 2 tablespoons olive oil
- 2 tablespoons reserved bean water
- ½ teaspoon sea salt
- Pinch ground cumin

Directions
1. With blender running, drop in a garlic clove to mince
2. Add remaining ingredients
3. Blitz until blended and creamy - additional bean water to your desired consistency.
4. Optional: top with dandelion "Gremolata" on page 142, pine nuts, and /or "Dukkah with Hemp" on page 135.

Cilantro Hummus

Ingredients
- 1-garlic clove
- 15-ounce can garbanzo beans drained - reserve bean water
- 1 bunch cilantro, remove thick stems at bottom of the bunch
- 2 tablespoons tahini
- 2 tablespoons olive oil
- 2 tablespoons fresh lime juice
- 2 tablespoons reserved bean water
- ½ teaspoon sea salt
- Pinch ground cumin
- Optional: Cilantro "Gremolata" on page 142 drizzled on top

Directions
1. With blender running, drop in a garlic clove to mince
2. Add the remaining ingredients: beans, cilantro, tahini, lime juice, olive oil, salt, and cumin.
3. Blitz until hummus is green, blended and creamy - add additional bean water to your desired consistency.

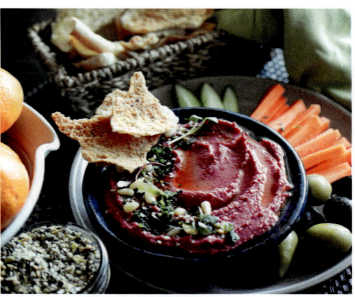

How to Roast Beet(s)

Ingredients
- 1 or more beets

Directions
1. Preheat oven to 350°F.
2. Remove green tops and scrub beet.
3. Wrap beet in foil.
4. Place on baking sheet and bake on center rack of oven for 60 minutes.
5. Remove from oven and cool until able to handle.
6. Remove from foil and remove skin.
7. Cut into pieces before adding to blender with other hummus ingredients.

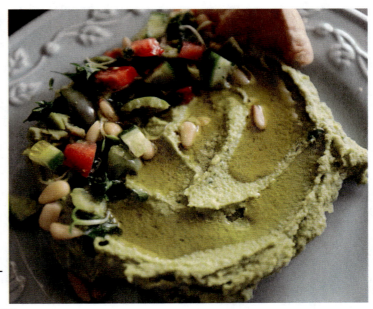

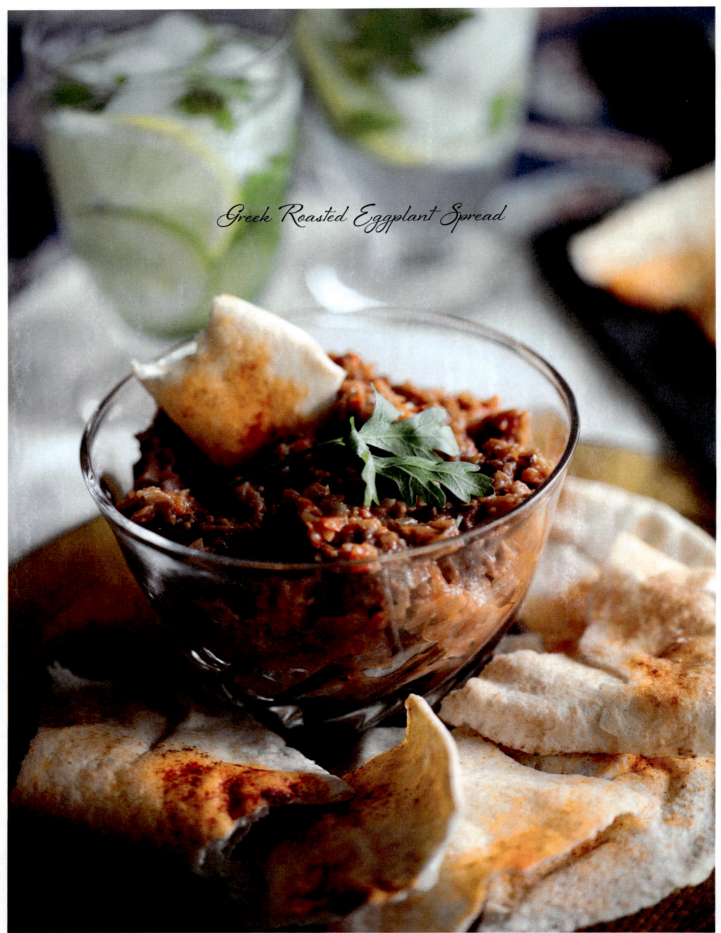
Greek Roasted Eggplant Spread

Greek Roasted Eggplant Spread

Makes approximately 1 pint sized jar of spread.

This eggplant spread makes an addictive addition to any mezze table. It even gets better the next day.

Ingredients

- 1 eggplant peeled diced
- 1 red bell pepper diced
- 1 sweet onion diced
- 1 garlic clove finely minced
- 2 tablespoons extra virgin olive oil
- 2 tablespoons tomato paste
- ¼ teaspoon cinnamon
- ¼ teaspoon ground oregano
- ¼ teaspoon sea salt or more to your taste
- Optional - flat Italian parsley finely chopped

Directions

1. Preheat oven to 400°F.
2. In a large bowl toss the eggplant, red bell pepper and onion pieces together with garlic, and olive oil.
3. Spread the veggies on a baking sheet lined with parchment paper.
4. Roast on the center rack of a 400°F preheated oven for 45 minutes or until soft, stirring once while cooking.
5. Remove roasted veggies from oven and place them in food processor fitted with a steel blade - add the tomato paste, cinnamon, ground oregano and salt - pulse about 10 times.
6. Spoon into serving dish with "Pita Chips" on page 52 or toasted slices of "Grilled Greek Toasts" on page 143, Italian or French bread.

Melitzanosalata

Eggplant Spread

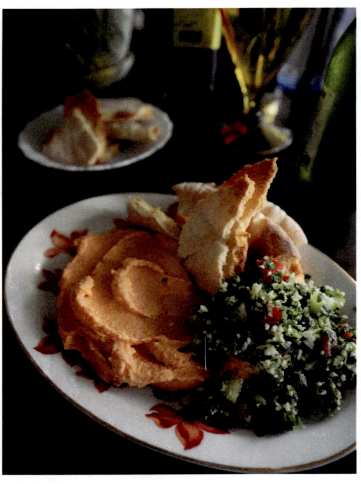

Roasted Red Bell Pepper Hummus

Ingredients

- 1-garlic clove
- 15-ounce can garbanzo beans drained - reserve bean water
- 1 roasted red bell pepper
- 2 tablespoons tahini
- 1 tablespoons fresh lemon juice
- 2 tablespoon olive oil
- ½ teaspoon sea salt
- Pinch ground cumin

Directions

1. With blender running, drop in a garlic clove to mince
2. Add the remaining ingredients: beans, bell pepper, tahini, lemon juice, olive oil, salt, and cumin.
3. Blitz until blended and creamy. Add bean water a tablespoon at a time for your desired consistency.

Raw Zucchini Hummus

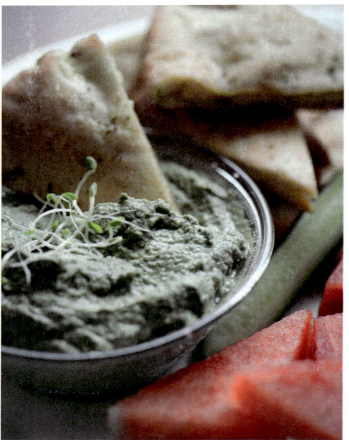

Ingredients

- 1-cup raw sunflower seeds soaked 4 hours or overnight
- 2 small zucchini unpeeled, coarsely chopped
- Juice of 1 lemon
- 2 garlic cloves minced
- ¼ cup raw tahini
- ½ teaspoon unrefined sea salt
- 1 tablespoon cold pressed extra virgin olive oil
- 1 small bunch cilantro

Directions

1. Drain and rinse sunflower seeds
2. Place all ingredients, except for cilantro, together in blender
3. Blitz on high until creamy
4. Add cilantro and pulse until blended in
5. Add additional water or olive oil for desired creaminess
6. Serve with veggies, "Pita Chips" on page 145 or "Grilled Greek Toasts" on page 143

Santorini Yellow Fava Hummus

A very common mezze born in the motherland of my ancestors, the Aegean islands. A light hummus made with yellow split peas.

Ingredients

- 1 cup dried yellow split peas
- 1 teaspoon unrefined sea salt divided
- 1 tablespoon sweet onion, finely minced
- 2 garlic cloves, finely minced
- 3 tablespoons extra virgin olive oil
- Juice of ½ lemon or more if you desire
- Chopped red onion and capers to garnish
- "Pita Chips" on page 145 for serving.

Directions

1. Rinse the split peas and place in a pot 4 cups of water with ½ teaspoon sea salt, and onion.
2. Bring to a boil over medium high heat, reduce heat to low and simmer uncovered for 25 to 30 minutes or until the water has been absorbed and split peas are soft— stir frequently.
3. Remove from stove and cool 15 minutes.
4. Add cooked split peas to blender along with remaining ½ teaspoon sea salt, garlic, olive oil, and lemon juice.
5. Process until mixture is smooth, scraping down sides of blender as needed.
6. Hummus will be less dense than chickpea hummus – and will firm up a little after cooled to room temperature.
7. Garnish with chopped red onion, chopped olives or capers, and additional olive oil.
8. Serve with Greek bread or pita chips.
9. Store in a glass jar with lid in refrigerator. Will keep for a week.

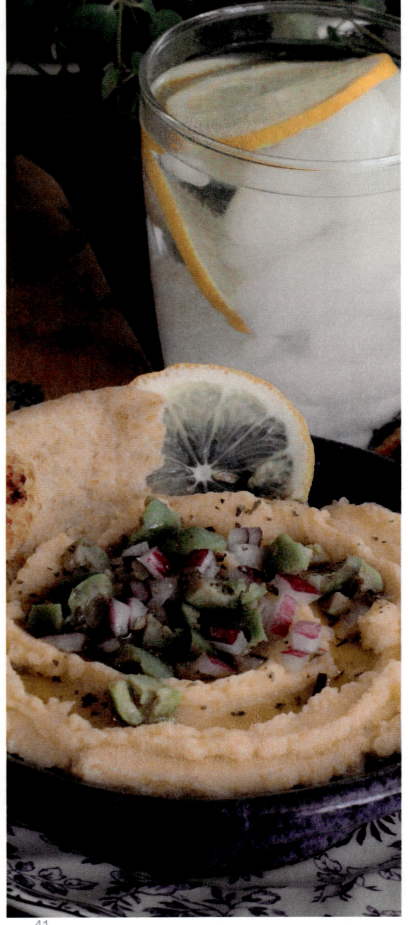

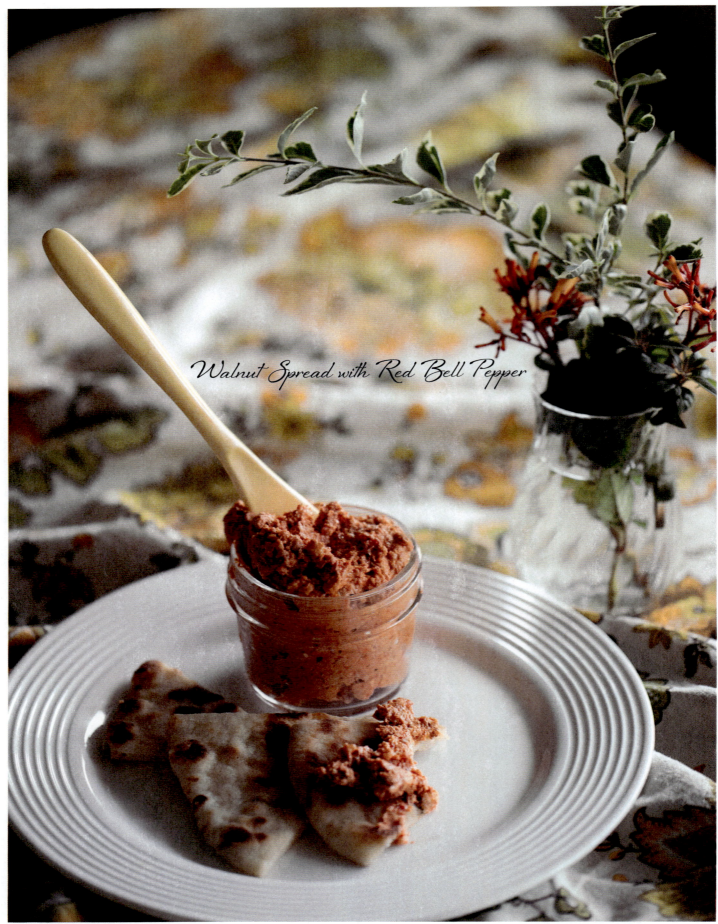
Walnut Spread with Red Bell Pepper

Walnut Spread

The day I made this wonderful Walnut Spread for photos, we had veggie burgers for dinner. I don't know why I didn't think of it sooner but...we used this spread as an additional condiment on our burgers. This elevated their tastiness to a heavenly realm of oh my yum!!! It satisfies the snacking spot when served on toasted pita - and packs flavor, nutrients, and protein as a dip for veggies.

Ingredients
- 1 garlic clove
- 1 red bell pepper from a jar, roasted
- ½ cup walnuts
- ¼ cup dried bread crumbs
- 1 tablespoon extra-virgin olive oil
- 1 teaspoon fresh lemon juice
- Unrefined sea salt to your taste

Directions
1. In a high-speed blender or food processor, drop garlic clove in with blender or processor running.
2. Add the red bell pepper, walnuts, bread crumbs, olive oil, and lemon juice.
3. Blitz ingredients together until blended.
4. Add water a tablespoon at a time if you prefer a thinner texture.
5. Add salt to your taste.

A la grecque

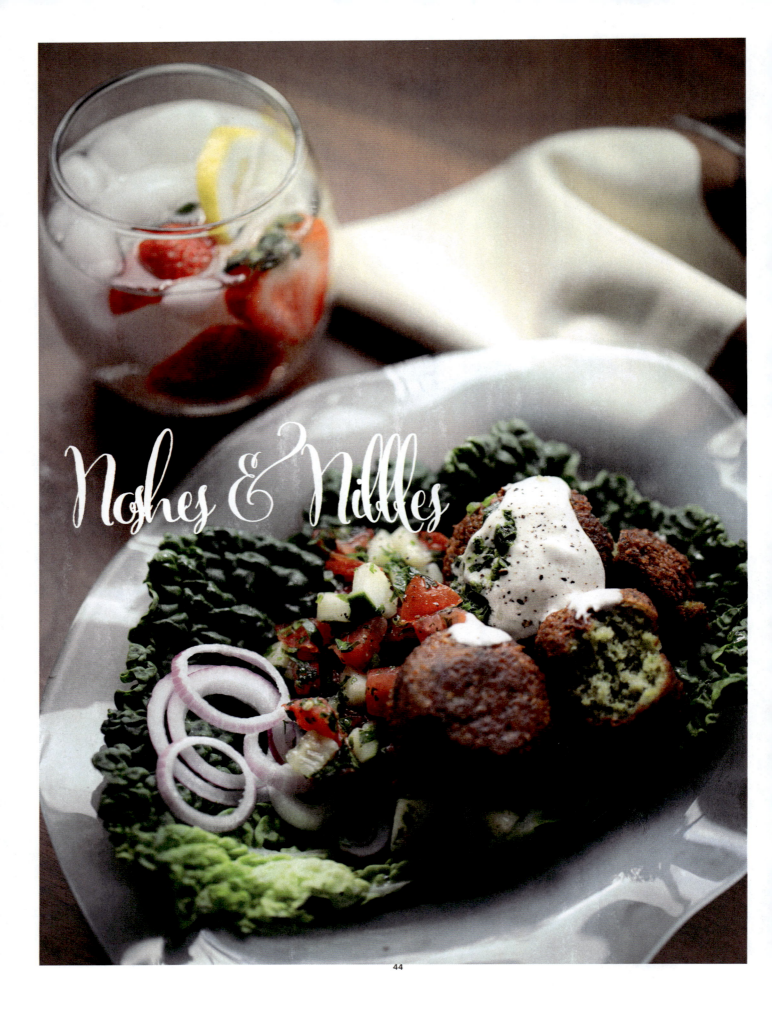

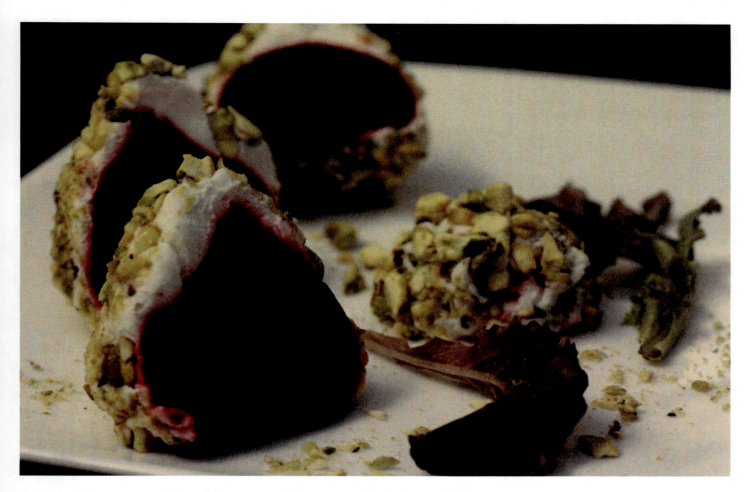

Baby Beets with Cream Cheese & Pistachios

This is a recipe I made for one of my final exams at Rouxbe Cooking School. These beets are beautiful, healthy, and delicious!

Ingredients

- 4 baby or very small beets roasted
- Non-dairy cream cheese, I like Kite Hill brand
- ¼ cup pistachios, finely chopped

Breathe properly. Stay curious. And eat your beets.

Tom Robbins

Directions

1. Preheat oven to 350° F.
2. Scrub beets, remove green tops, wrap in foil.
3. Bake in preheated oven for 45 to 60 minutes or until tender when pierced with a knife.
4. Remove from oven, cool, and peel.
5. Cut thin slice off of bottom of beets to help them stand, and pat them dry.
6. Let cream cheese sit at room temp. for 15 minutes to soften.
7. Press a little cream cheese onto beets.
8. Roll and press the beets into pistachios.
9. Cut beets into halves.
10. Serve chilled.

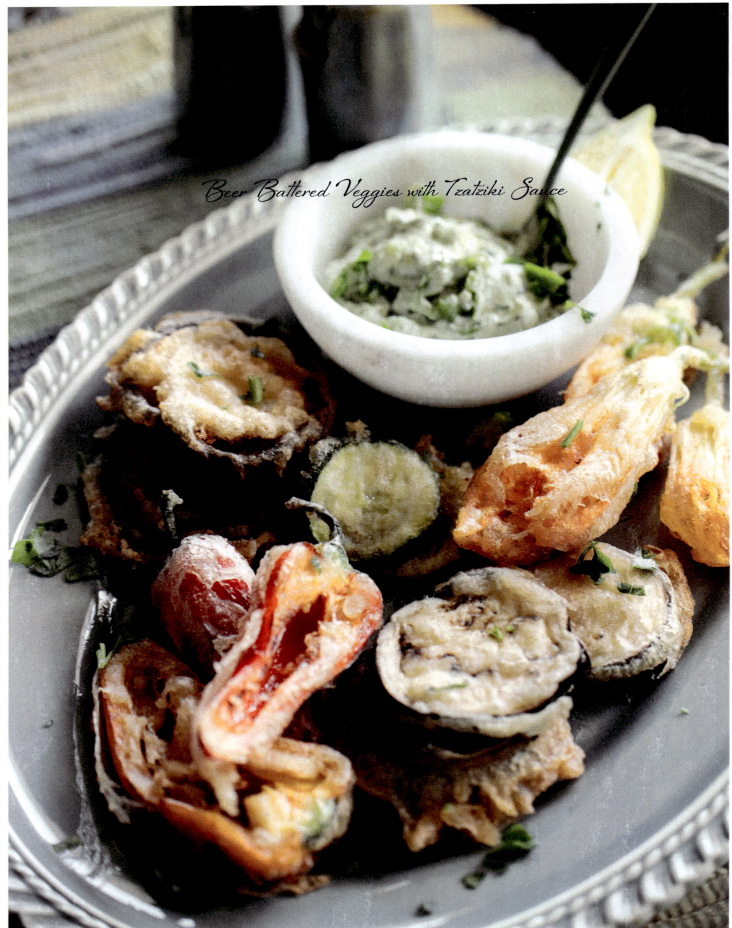

Beer Battered Veggies with Tzatziki Sauce

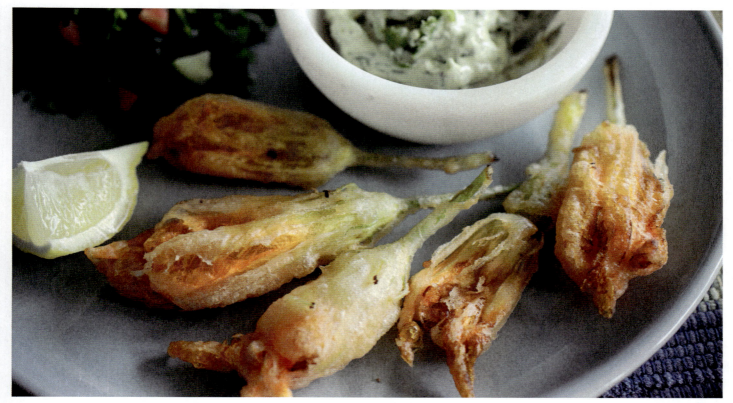

Zucchini Blossoms Fried in Beer Batter

Beer Batter Recipe

A sure way to increase my family's veggie intake is by occasionally shallow frying. I only use extra light olive oil and only in small amounts over medium to medium-low heat. Research shows veggies fried in olive oil have valuable micronutrients and phytochemicals. I use a thin beer batter and avoid heavy breading. I also have a secret ingredient that keeps the veggies crispy. It's rice flour. Rice flour is available at some large grocery stores or from Asian markets.

Because mezzes are small bites, it's nice to have a guilt-free taste of delicious of crispy fried veggies – especially in the spring when the squash blossoms are in bloom.

Ingredients

- ¾ cup all-purpose flour
- ¼ cup rice flour
- ½ teaspoon baking powder
- ½ teaspoon garlic powder
- ¼ teaspoon paprika
- ¼ teaspoon unrefined sea salt
- ¾ cup cold beer – Budweiser beer and Mythos Greek beer are plant-based friendly
- Extra light olive oil

Directions

1. Whisk all-purpose flour, rice flour, baking powder, garlic powder, paprika, and salt, together in a medium bowl.
2. Reserve ¼ cup of the dry mixture to toss with veggies.
3. Slice zucchini and eggplant
4. Heat oil in medium skillet over medium low heat.
5. Whisk cold beer into the remaining flour mixture. Your batter should be thin. Add an ice cube to keep the mixture cool.
6. Fry veggies in beer batter as directed by the recipe.

Beer Battered Blossoms & Veggies

Fritto Misto

Use your favorite veggie or veggies for this recipe.

Ingredients

- Small eggplant cut into ½ inch slices
- 1 zucchini cut into ½ inch slices
- Unrefined sea salt
- Button mushrooms, left whole
- Mini sweet peppers, cut in half
- Squash blossoms
- Extra light olive oil for frying
- "Tzatziki Dressing" on page 33
- Lemon wedges
- 1 recipe "Beer Batter Recipe" on page 47 - reserve 1/4 cup of dry mixture before adding beer to coat veggies before frying

Variety is the Spice of Life

Veggie Directions

1. Sprinkle salt on eggplant and zucchini slices – place slices in colander to drain for 30 minutes.
2. Rinse eggplant and zucchini to remove salt - pat and gently press dry with paper towels.
3. Very gently rinse blossoms and gently pat dry.
4. In large bowl, toss veggies with reserved DRY mixture from beer batter – be especially gentle with blossoms.
5. Pour 1/2 inch of olive oil into skillet on medium heat.
6. Test oil before frying by dropping a drip of batter into skillet - it should sizzle.
7. Working in batches, dip veggies into beer batter – drain off extra batter - you only want a very thin layer of batter on veggies - fry blossoms last.
8. Carefully place battered veggies into hot oil.
9. Shallow fry in oil for 2 to 3 minutes on each side or until lightly crisp and golden.
10. Drain on paper towels.
11. Dip blossoms into batter and gently remove excess batter with fingers
12. Fry 1 to 2 minutes on each side turning once.
13. Drain on paper towels.
14. Serve immediately with lemon wedges and optional Tzatziki Dressing.

Beer Battered "Cardoona"

I cooked for a small community of Franciscan Friars for almost 16-years. Most of the friars were Italian. I loved to listen to their stories about their family's favorite foods. That's how I learned about "cardoona." The Guardian, Fr. Peter, told me his family felt like they hit the jackpot when they discovered a secret patch of wild cardoon a few yards off a country road in Sicily. He said each spring they looked forward to foraging all the "cardoona" they could possibly eat.

Cardoons are a cousin of the artichoke family. They look like large stalks of pale green, velvet celery. They have the crunch of celery with a faint floral taste of artichoke. The friars' families would add cardoons to soups and stews – and pickle the surplus. But their all-time favorite way to enjoy this uncommon veggie was pan-fried in a light batter.

I've personally never seen cardoons in a chain grocery store. Still, they can be found in Italian or Mediterranean markets around St. Joseph's Feast Day, March 19th. In honor of the season and the saint, little old Italian ladies of the parish would bring warm fried cardoons as gifts to the friars. The friars would gather to graze on the crispy green stalks and reminisce about their "cardoona" encounters from their younger years.

When cardoons are in season, you've got to get to the market early. They're an Italian delicacy and disappear soon after they're placed on the shelf. When I saw a bunch at the market this morning - I snatched them up to serve as a mezze and to share my own cardoon stories from the friary. They are delicious sprinkled with a little coarse salt. But they're downright addictive when served as a sweet - pressed in a little cane or confectioners' sugar.

Ingredients

- 1/2 to 1 bunch of cardoon ribs - the bunches can sometimes be large
- "Beer Batter Recipe" on page 47
- Extra light olive oil for frying
- Optional: coarse finishing salt (like Chion or French Maldon) or raw cane or confectioners' sugar.

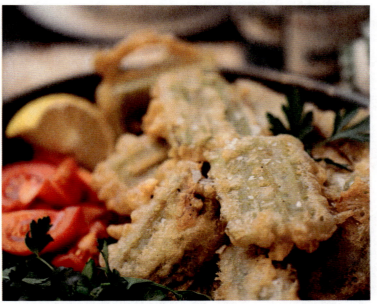

Directions

1. Separate the cardoon stalks and thoroughly wash.
2. Trim the bottoms and remove any leaves.
3. Cut the ribs into 2-inch pieces
4. Bring a medium pot of water to a boil over medium heat.
5. Add the cardoon pieces to the boiling water, reduce heat and simmer for 10 minutes uncovered.
6. Transfer to a colander and drain well - cool to room temperature.
7. Lightly press pieces with paper towel to remove additional moisture and place in medium bowl.
8. Toss with ¼ cup of the dry Beer Batter ingredients to coat.
9. Add cardoon pieces to the Beer Batter.
10. Heat ½ inch of olive oil in large skillet over medium heat.
11. Carefully drop pieces of battered cardoons into hot oil – work in batches – do not crowd while frying.
12. Cook for 5 to 7 minutes or until lightly golden brown.
13. Transfer to paper towels.
14. Sprinkle with coarse salt or press into raw cane sugar.
15. Best if served immediately.

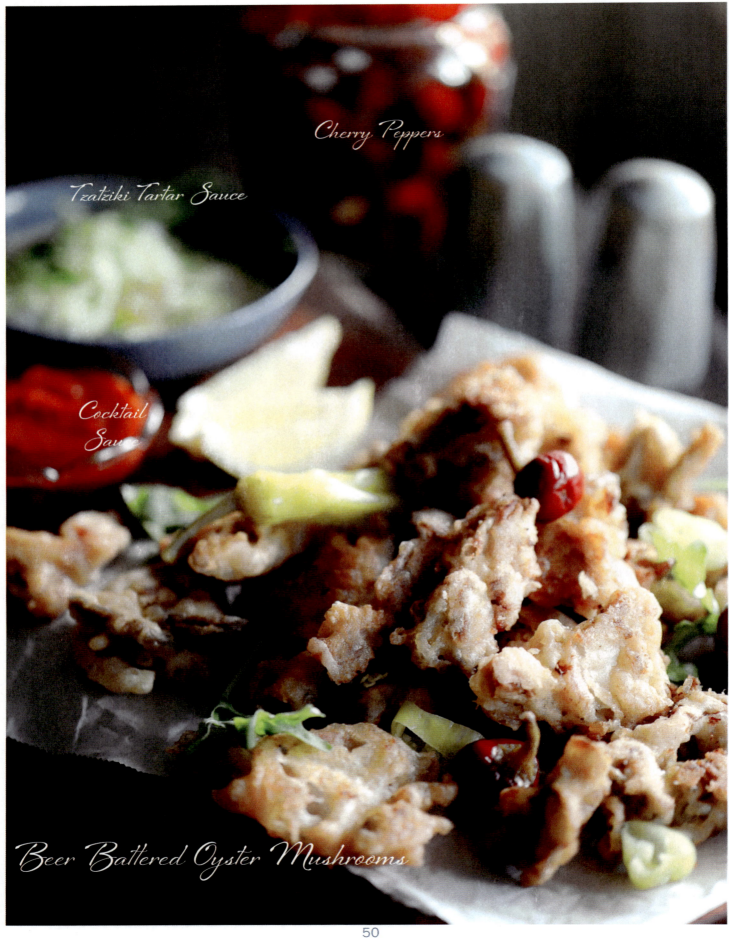

Beer Battered Oysters

Makes 6 to 12 mezze portions.

I use oyster mushrooms for this family favorite mezze. I find them at the Asian grocery store. Beer batter adds depth of flavor and crispiness to these yummy oysters.

Ingredients

- Approximately 1 pound oyster mushrooms
- Extra light olive oil for shallow frying
- "Beer Batter Recipe" on page 47
- "Tzatziki Tartar Sauce" see below
- Optional: serve with lemon wedges, sliced Greek peppers, & cherry peppers

Oyster Mushroom Directions

1. Oyster mushroom grow on a mushroom base. Pull or cut the mushrooms from the base – they should approximate the size of oysters.
2. Rinse thoroughly and drain in a colander.
3. While mushrooms are draining, make the beer batter.
4. In a medium bowl whisk together the all-purpose flour, rice flour, baking powder, garlic powder, paprika, and salt.
5. Reserve ¼ cup of the dry mixture.
6. Pat the mushrooms dry with paper towels.
7. In a skillet, heat ½ inch of oil over medium heat. Because the mushrooms are not meat, they cook faster and do not need to be submerged in hot oil.
8. Toss the mushrooms to coat with the ¼ cup of reserved flour mix.
9. Whisk beer into remaining flour mixture – mixture should not be too thick but the consistency of heavy cream.
10. Test the oil – it should sizzle when you drop in a drop of batter.
11. Dip each mushroom oyster into the beer batter. Allow excess batter to drain off.
12. Carefully place mushrooms in the oil and fry for 2 to 3 minutes – turning half way through cooking until they are evenly browned.
13. Remove cooked oysters from oil and drain on paper towels.
14. Do not over crowd the mushrooms – cook in batches.
15. Serve immediately with Tzatziki Tartar Sauce, cocktail sauce, lemon wedges, cherry peppers, and sliced Greek peppers.

Greek Oyster Po Boy

1. Serve fried oysters on small warmed pitas with Tzatziki Sauce, shredded lettuce, sliced dill pickles, and sliced grape tomatoes..
2. Sprinkle with a little dried oregano.
3. Serve immediately.

Tzatziki Tartar Sauce

Add 1 tablespoon sweet pickle relish to "Tzatziki Dressing" on page 33

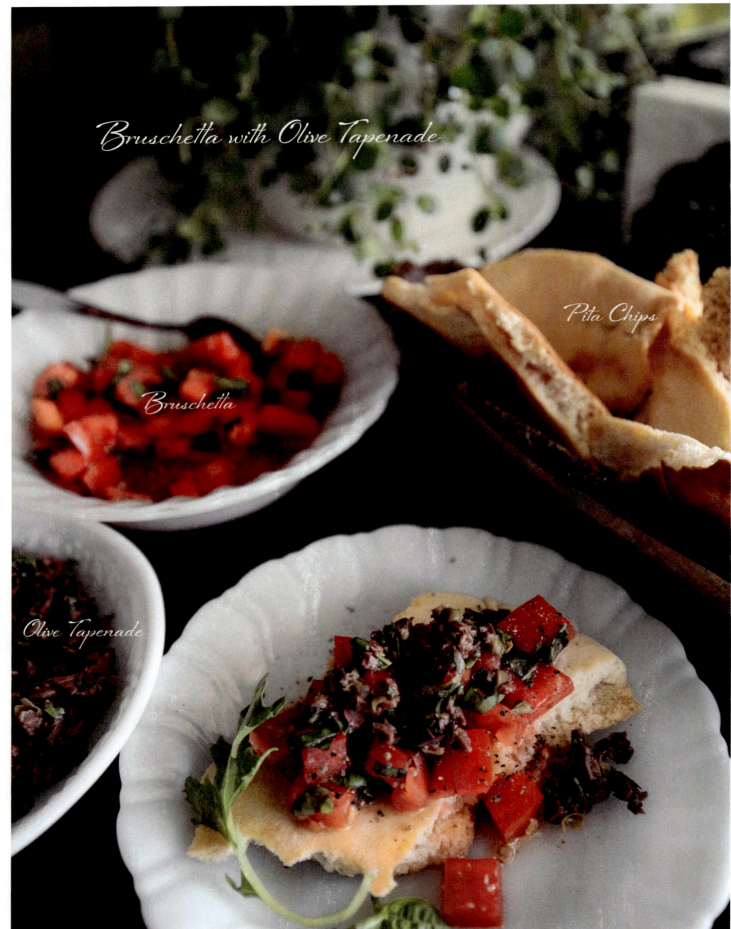

Bruschetta Greek Style

Makes 8 servings

Ingredients

- 4 Roma or plum tomatoes diced into small cubes
- ½ teaspoon unrefined sea salt
- 3 tablespoons extra virgin olive oil
- 2 garlic cloves finely minced
- 8 fresh basil leaves chopped
- "Olive Tapenade" on page 55
- Pita chips or grilled slices of Greek bread

Directions

1. In small bowl toss diced tomatoes with salt.
2. In small skillet heat olive oil with garlic over low heat for 5 minutes, stirring frequently to keep the garlic from turning brown.
3. Cool garlic and olive oil to room temperature.
4. Add garlic and olive oil to tomatoes.
5. Layer basil leaves on top of each other and roll up – cut roll into fine strips then chop.
6. Toss chopped basil leaves with tomatoes.
7. Serve tomatoes on "Pita Chips" on page 145 or "Grilled Greek Toasts" on page 143
8. Top Bruschetta tomatoes with "Olive Tapenade" on page 55

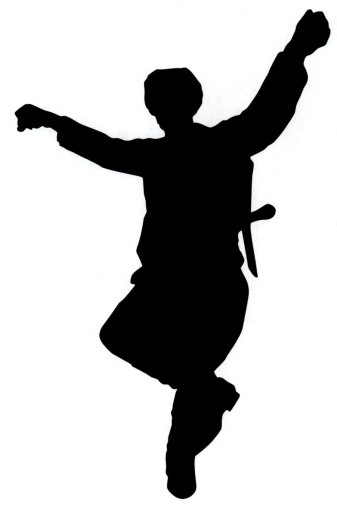

Apolamvano!
Enjoy!

Fast Food

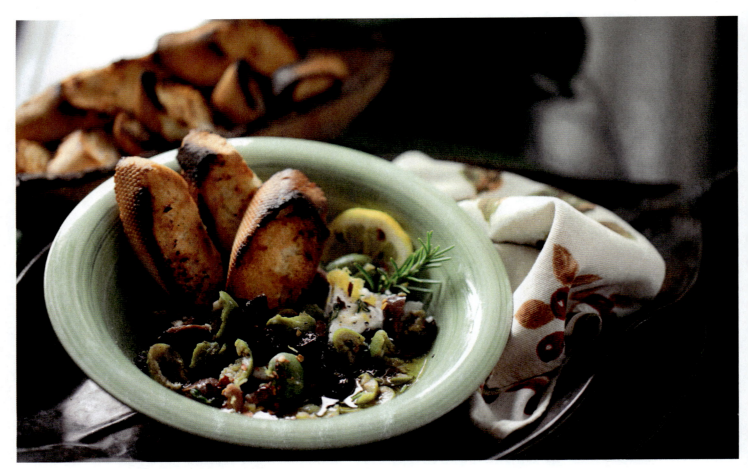

Cracked Marinated Olives

Makes 6 to 8 mezze servings.

"The olive tree is surely the richest gift of Heaven."

Thomas Jefferson

Tarpon Springs was a wonderful and safe place to grow up. I used to walk a mile to and from elementary school with family and other kids in the neighborhood. Even as a child, my Greek foodie genes were expressing themselves. Along the way home from school, we would pass a small, 2-story, wooden house whose downstairs was a Greek deli; the owners lived upstairs. A couple of times a week, we would make a stop at this little store. Most of the kids, including my family members, would buy candy – like Red Hots, Milk Duds, Candy Cigarettes, etc. I remember fighting back embarrassment and summoning up the courage to spend my pennies on olives and feta. The deli server and I had a soul-food connection. He always winked and smiled as he handed me a small white paper container with a couple of olives and a dice-sized cube of white cheese. My kid companions mocked me, but savoring the black, briny fruits and creamy feta was worth every "eww".

I like to use a pint of assorted olives from an olive bar at a local Mediterranean market to make this recipe. This olive recipe is briny and lemony with a hint of heat. They make a mouthwatering appetizer to serve at a mezze get-together. I also like to use olives with pits, and remove the pits myself. I don't understand it, but to me, olives with pits are much more flavorful. Do a taste test - see if you agree.

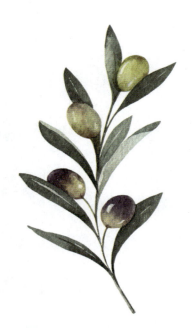

Ingredients Cracked Marinated olives

- 1- pint assorted olives with pits
- 1 garlic clove minced
- Lemon zest from 1 organic lemon
- Fresh lemon juice from ½ organic lemon, slice the remaining lemon half
- 3 sprigs fresh rosemary chopped
- 1/4 teaspoon red pepper flakes
- 1/4 teaspoon dried oregano
- A few grinds of fresh pepper
- Pinch of sea salt
- Optional plant-based feta
- "Pita Chips" on page 145 or "Grilled Greek Toasts" on page 143

Directions

I buy olives with the pits intact. They are plumper and more flavorful. Use a chef's knife to press the olives against a cutting board until they crack open. Remove the seeds and proceed with the recipe.

1. Remove seeds from olives and coarsely chop.
2. Mix the olives, garlic, lemon zest, rosemary, red pepper flakes, oregano, pepper, and sea salt together in a small bowl..
3. Serve with pita chips or grilled slices of bread and a little plant-based feta.
4. Olive oil solidifies when refrigerated so this recipe is best served at room temperature.

Olive Tapenade

Makes 1 pint tapenade

Directions

1. Use the recipe ingredients for Cracked Marinated Olives.
2. Remove seeds from olives.
3. Using a chef's knife, finely chop the olives.
4. In small bowl, mix the finely chopped olives with the garlic, lemon zest, lemon juice, rosemary, red pepper flakes, oregano, pepper, and sea salt.
5. Optional: toss in 2 tablespoons finely chopped curly parsley.
6. Serve with "Pita Chips" on page 145 or "Grilled Greek Toasts" on page 143

Ways to use Olive Tapenade

- As a topping for hummus
- To stuff celery or grape tomatoes
- Sprinkle on pizza
- Use as a spread on sandwiches or veggie burgers
- As a topping on bruschetta
- As a topping on avocado toast
- Use your imagination

Kali Orexi

Bon Appetite

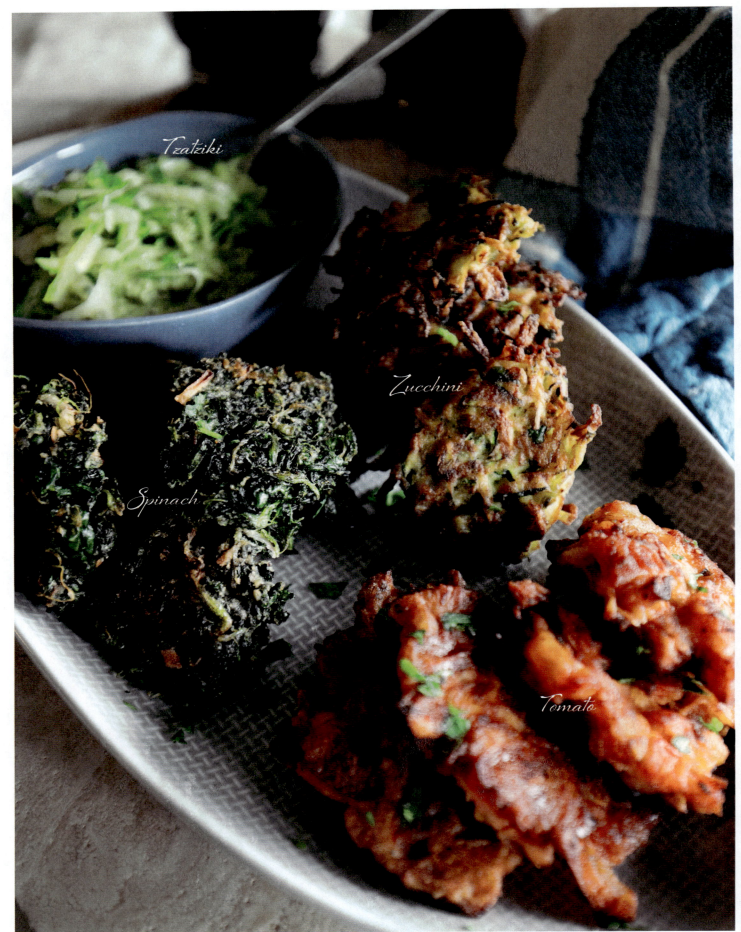

Veggie Fritters

Nostalgia has a way of rehabbing humble foods into esteemed eatables. In my kitchen, fritters have evolved from meh to marvelous. Fritters are not only a homey taste from my childhood, but they're also a satisfying way to expand my plant-based treasure-trove. I took lessons from my mother's kitchen and built on them. My fritters are just as yummy but are easier and healthier. I replaced white, all-purpose flour with garbanzo bean flour – and I only use just enough to bind the veggies. Garbanzo bean flour adds protein, fiber, and micronutrients to the recipe. Liquid from the veggies, and not eggs, form the batter. Instead of deep-frying, I shallow-fry my fritters in health-giving olive oil. Because my fritters are small and less dense than my mothers, alternating medium to medium-low heat is just hot enough to produce golden brown patties without leaving them oily.

Zucchini Fritters

Yield – approximately 12 fritters

Ingredients

- 2 medium zucchinis, shredded
- ½ cup sweet onion coarsely chopped
- 1 garlic clove finely minced
- 2 teaspoons dried mint
- ½ teaspoon dried oregano
- ¼ teaspoon salt
- ½ cup garbanzo bean flour
- Olive oil for frying

Directions

1. To medium bowl, add zucchini, garlic onion, mint, oregano, and salt – toss to blend ingredients.
2. Add garbanzo bean flour – I like to mix in the flour using my hands.
3. Mixture will be a little wet but should not be watery – add small amounts of flour if needed.
4. Allow the fritter mixture to rest for 10 minutes.
5. Heat skillet over medium heat.
6. Pour about ¼ inch of olive oil into preheated skillet.
7. Drop tablespoons full of fritter mixture onto the hot oil and fry for 2 to 3 minutes on each side – if fritters seem to brown too quickly, reduce heat to medium low.
8. Fritters should be golden brown and not greasy.
9. Transfer to paper towel lined plate.
10. Best if served immediately with Tzatziki or vegan sour cream.

Spinach Fritters

Yield approximately 12 fritters

Ingredients

- 16-ounce frozen chopped spinach thawed
- ½ sweet onion finely chopped
- 1 teaspoon dried dill
- 1 teaspoon dried mint
- ¼ teaspoon salt
- ½ cup garbanzo bean flour

Directions

1. Press water out of spinach and place in a medium bowl
2. Add onion, dill, mint, salt and garbanzo bean flour
3. Follow directions for Zucchini Fritters.

Tomato Fritters

Yield approximately 12 fritters

Ingredients

- 3 Roma tomatoes cut into small cubes
- 1 shallot finely minced
- ¼ teaspoon salt
- ½ teaspoon dried oregano
- ½ teaspoon dried mint
- ½ cup garbanzo bean flour, plus more as needed
- Extra Light Olive oil for frying

Directions

1. Follow directions as written for zucchini fritters – but tomato fritters burn more easily, fry on a medium-low heat.

Green Falafels

Falafels were on the menu at Saint Francis Cafe. When a girl from Israel visited, she told us our falafel sandwich was the best she ever tasted. In addition to falafels wrapped with a veggie leaf, we also served them on warm pita, on our Greek salad or just for dipping in tzatziki or tahini dressing. This recipe makes approximately 24 delicious mezze-sized falafel balls.

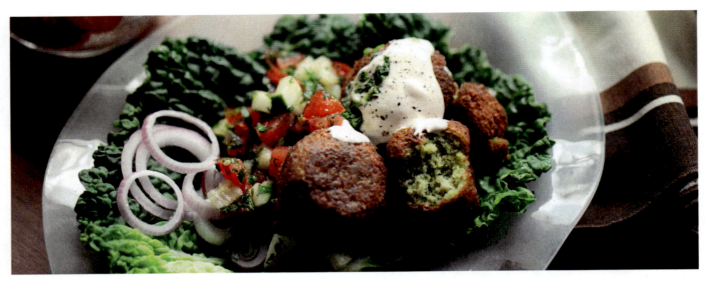

Ingredients

- 16-ounce package dried chickpeas soaked overnight
- 3 garlic cloves
- 1 large bunch (or 2 small bunches) cilantro
- 1 white onion, coarsely chopped
- 2 teaspoons sea salt
- ½ teaspoon ground coriander
- 1/8-teaspoon cumin
- 1-teaspoon baking powder
- ¼ cup bread flour
- Extra-light olive oil for frying
- Tahini Dressing

Directions

1. Pick over and wash the chickpeas.
2. Place in bowl and cover with 3 inches of filtered water and soak overnight at room temperature.
3. Rinse the soaked beans and drain well.
4. With food processor running, drop in garlic cloves to mince.
5. To food processor bowl, add chickpeas, cilantro, onion, sea salt, coriander and cumin - pulse until finely minced to form a paste.
6. Remove from processor – stir in baking powder and flour.
7. Cover and refrigerate 3 to 4 hours for flavors to blend.
8. Heat 1/2 inch of oil over medium heat in large skillet.
9. If the falafel mixture is too loose add a little more flour just until the falafel holds together to form a ball.
10. Using small ice-cream scoop to scoop up falafel mixture and drop into oil - or roll a tablespoon of mixture in between palms to form a ball and carefully drop into oil.
11. Shallow fry approximately 3 minutes or until golden brown – turning with a slotted spoon as needed to cook through and brown on all sides.
12. Remove with slotted spoon and place on paper-towel to blot excess oil.
13. Make a small green falafel sliders by serving on a green leaf of lettuce or kale - top with "Tabouli with Celery & Mint" on page 25 or diced tomatoes, cucumber, sliced onion and "Tahini Dressing" on page 33.
14. Or - serve with falafels on a mezze platter with Tahini Dressing and/or on a "Greek Salad" on page 12.
15. Or - make a falafel slider. Make falafel patties. Serve on a small toasted bun, with grilled onion, tomato, cucumber, lettuce, & "Tzatziki Dressing" on page 33i.

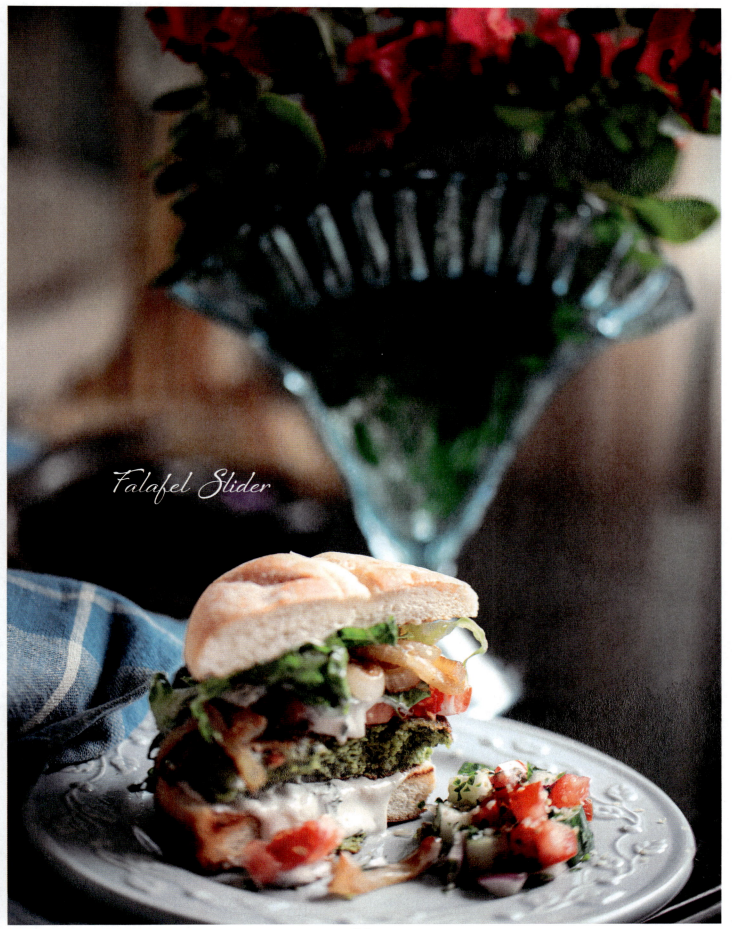
Falafel Slider

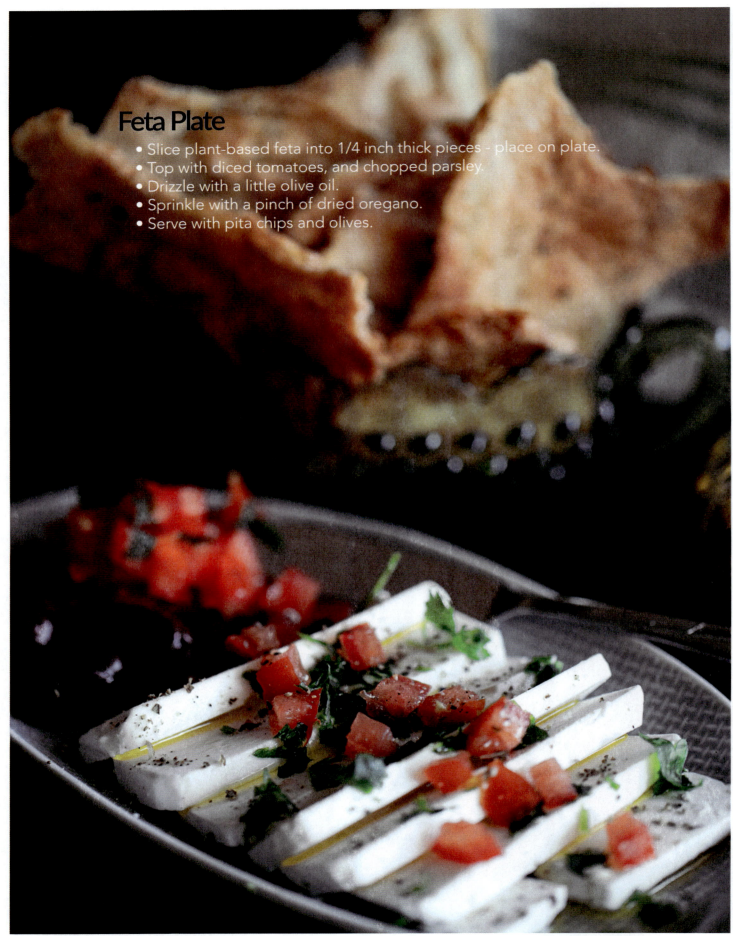

Feta Plate

- Slice plant-based feta into 1/4 inch thick pieces - place on plate.
- Top with diced tomatoes, and chopped parsley.
- Drizzle with a little olive oil.
- Sprinkle with a pinch of dried oregano.
- Serve with pita chips and olives.

Greek Gazpacho

Makes 4 mezze-sized servings.

Juicy, vine-ripened tomatoes are on my list of profoundly satisfying comfort foods. We had tomatoes at most evening meals – we dined on them in salads, soups, and entrees. Occasionally, my father tossed chopped tomatoes with scrambled eggs for breakfast. For lunch, we enjoyed thick slices, salted and stacked on soft Greek bread generously slathered with creamy mayo. But my fondest tomato memory was an after-dinner ritual. I would slurp up the briny tomato juices left behind from a salad in the bottom of our family's cherished wooden salad bowl. The bowl was brought to America by yia yia from her birth island, Symi. Because my mother found slurping highly offensive, I sipped the tomato liquor with dressing - alone in abandon on the back porch. The lesson in this story is - those mouthwatering moments of transcendent slabber were the inspiration for my Greek Gazpacho.

Ingredients

- 1 pint grape tomatoes
- 4 Kalamata olives, seeded
- 1 generous pinch from a bunch of flat Italian parsley
- 1/2-teaspoon fresh lemon juice
- 1-teaspoon apple cider vinegar
- 1/2-teaspoon dried oregano
- 1-teaspoon olive oil
- A splash or 2 of cold water
- Salt and fresh cracked pepper to taste
- Additional Kalamata olives chopped for garnish

Directions

1. Place tomatoes together with olives, parsley, lemon juice, vinegar, oregano and olive oil in the blender.
2. Pulse until combined but slightly chunky.
3. Add a few splashes of cold water for desired consistency.
4. Unrefined sea salt and fresh milled pepper to your taste.
5. Serve garnished with additional chopped olives and a tiny pinch of dried oregano

Fresh!

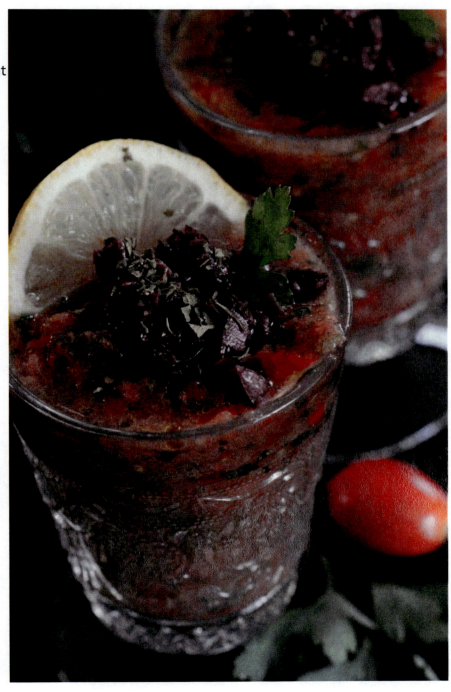

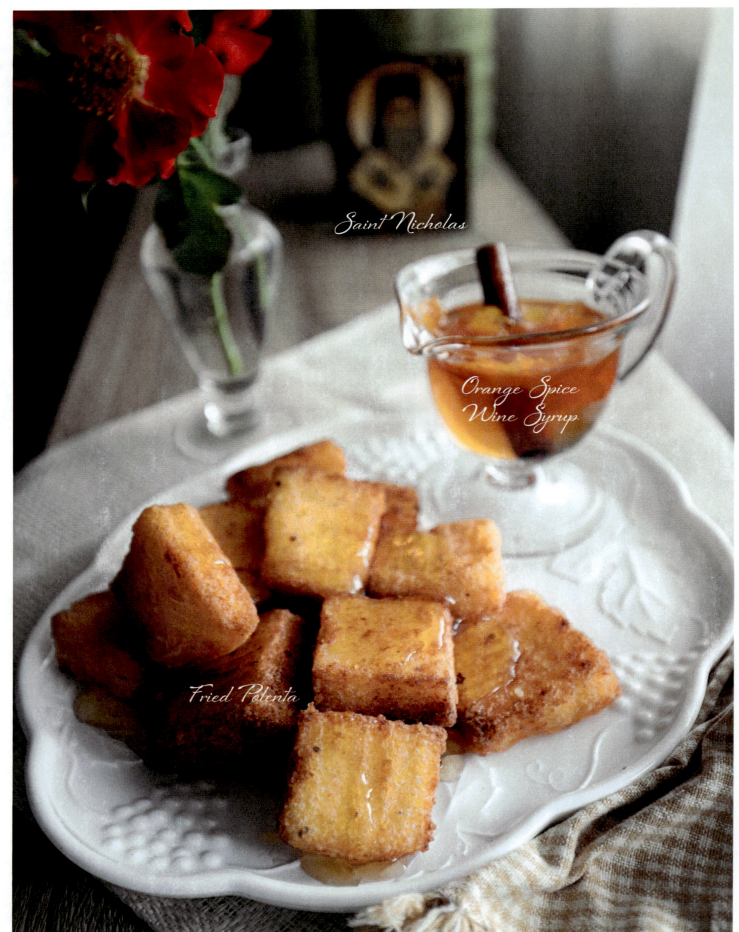

Fried Polenta

Yield 12 to 16 mezze squares.

My mother often made white corn grits for breakfast. She would serve them like a thick porridge. We ate them with a little salt and butter or cream and sugar. She poured warm leftovers onto a piece of waxed paper, and they solidified as they cooled. She would cut the cooled slab into squares then crisp them in a frying pan with a little oil. She served them plain or with a side of honey as a special treat.

I also prepared white grits for my family until I learned about polenta from the friars. Italian polenta, aka yellow grits, are unbleached, less processed, and far more flavorful. When I fry Italian polenta, my family stays close to the kitchen. This way, they can snatch a crispy polenta square right as it comes out of the frying pan - many times, they disappear before I can get them to the table.

Shallow fried Italian polenta squares make a delicious mezze. Add a little Orange Spice Syrup, Tomato Jam, or Schug - now you have an exceptionally tasty, and addictive mezze.

The uncooked polenta slab can stay covered in the refrigerator for 3 to 4 days. Just before serving, I shallow fry the polenta squares in a little extra light olive oil until crisp. Warning! Keep a close watch for crispy polenta square thieves.

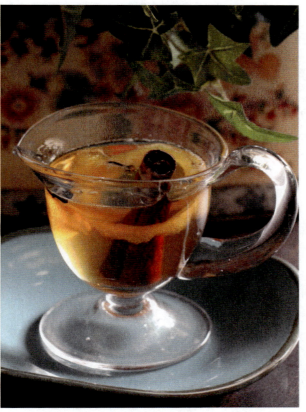

Orange Spice Wine Syrup

Ingredients

- 3 cups filtered or spring water
- ½ teaspoon salt
- 1-cup polenta – I love Bob's Red Mill Organic Polenta, hands down the best!
- Optional – 2 tablespoons vegan butter
- All purpose flour to coat the squares
- Extra light olive oil for frying

Directions

1. In small saucepan bring water and salt to a boil over high heat.
2. Slowly whisk in polenta and reduce heat to low.
3. Continue to cook, whisking frequently, for about 15 to 30 minutes or until polenta becomes cooked through and creamy.
4. Remove from stove and spoon onto parchment lined baking sheet and spread with spatula to an even thickness rectangle – about ¾ of an inch.
5. Once thoroughly cooled, cut the polenta slab into 1-inch squares and refrigerate 1 hour or overnight.
6. In medium frying pan heat ¼ inch deep oil over medium heat.
7. Put a little all purpose flour in a pie plate or shallow bowl.
8. Dust polenta squares with a little flour patting and shaking off any excess.
9. Carefully place squares into hot oil and cook until golden brown on both sides, about 2 to 3 minutes per side.
10. Adjust the medium heat to medium low as needed to keep polenta squares from burning.
11. Drain on paper towels.
12. Serve immediately plain, with"Orange Spiced Wine Syrup" on page 144.

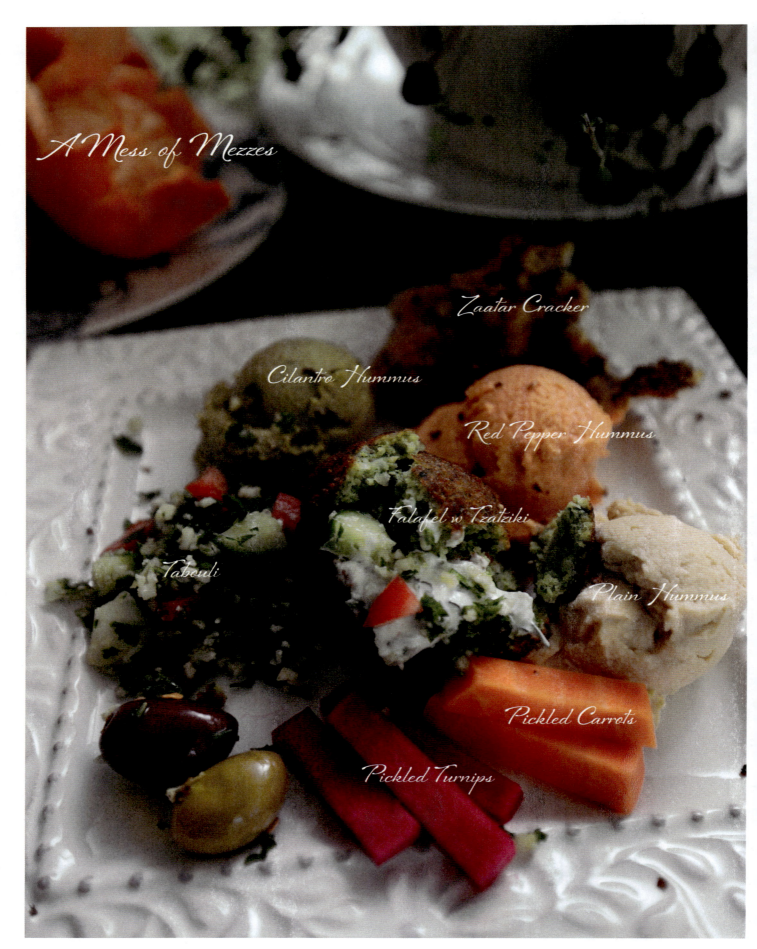

Greek Guac

If you have nothing but love for your avocados, and you take joy in turning them into guacamole, all you need is someone to share it with.

Jason Mraz

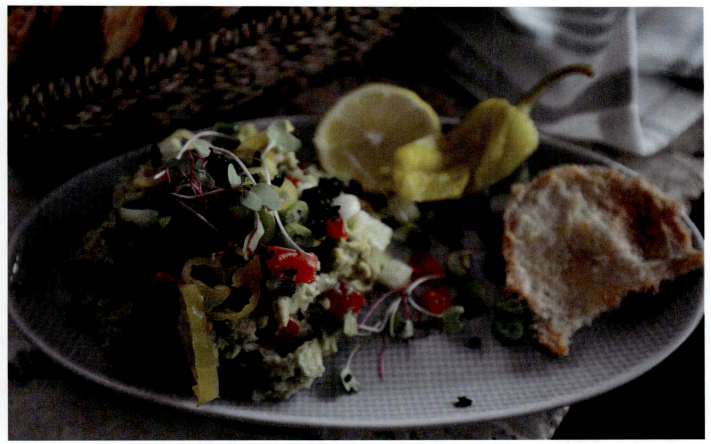

Ingredients

- 2 Haas avocados, peeled and seeds removed
- 2 teaspoons fresh lemon juice
- 1 tablespoon Kalamata or Greek black olives finely chopped
- 2 Campari or 2 Roma tomatoes seeded and diced
- 1 small Persian cucumber with skin, diced into small cubes.
- 1 green onion with green parts finely sliced
- 1 Greek pepperoncini, thinly sliced and 1 for garnish
- Optional: ½ teaspoon Greek Seasoning Blend or dried oregano
- Unrefined sea salt to your desired taste
- Microgreens for additional superfood antioxidants and other nutrients

Directions

1. Wash the avocados, cut them into halves, remove seed.
2. Using a spoon, scoop the flesh out into small bowl.
3. Coarsely mash the avocado with 2 teaspoons of lemon juice using a fork.
4. Gently stir in chopped olives, tomatoes, cucumber, green onion, pepperoncini, "Greek Seasoning Blend" on page 142.
5. If desired, add a little sea salt.
6. Serve on mezze table with pita break or "Pita Chips" on page 145.
7. Sprinkle with microgreens.
8. Best if eaten on same day.

Fruit Plate

Placing seasonal fruits on a plate makes a simple and beautiful mezze offering. Add a few almonds or walnuts for plant-based protein.

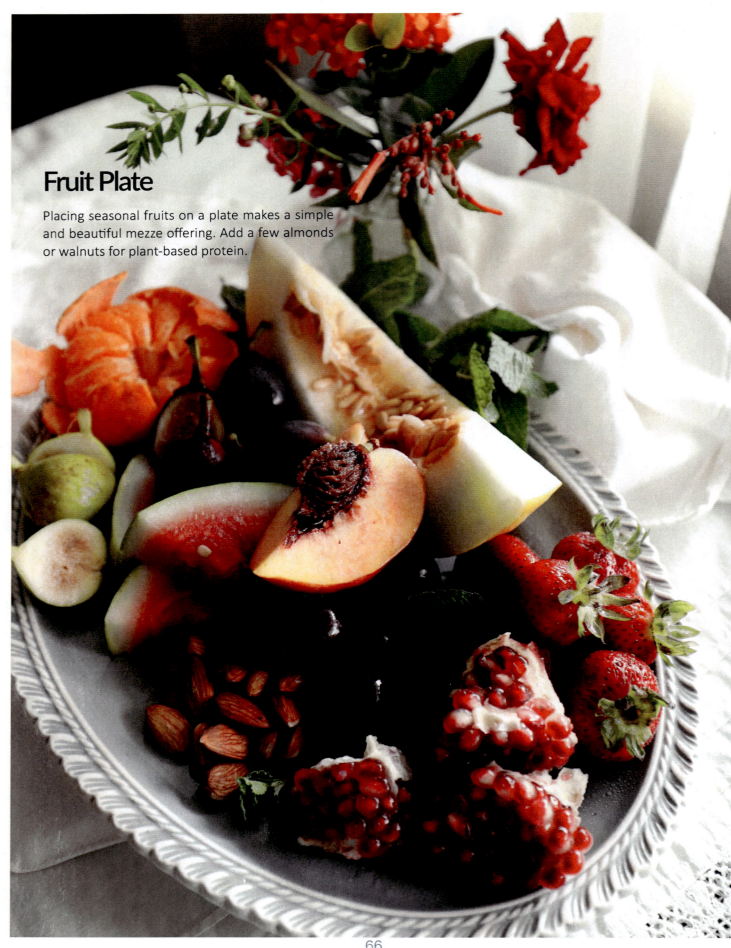

All you need is love – and a veggie platter...

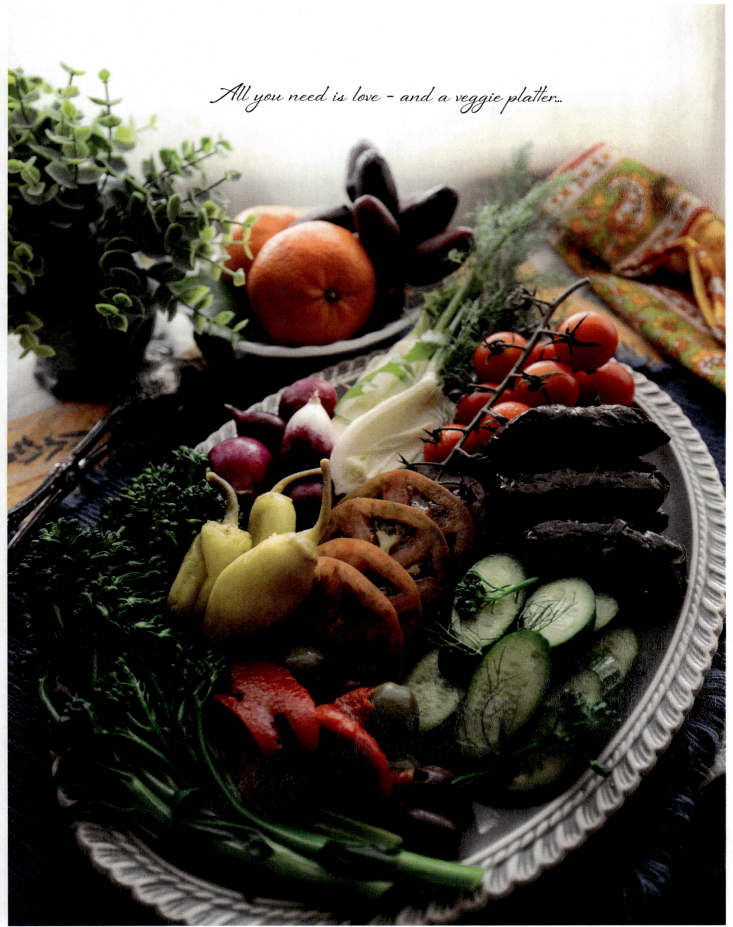

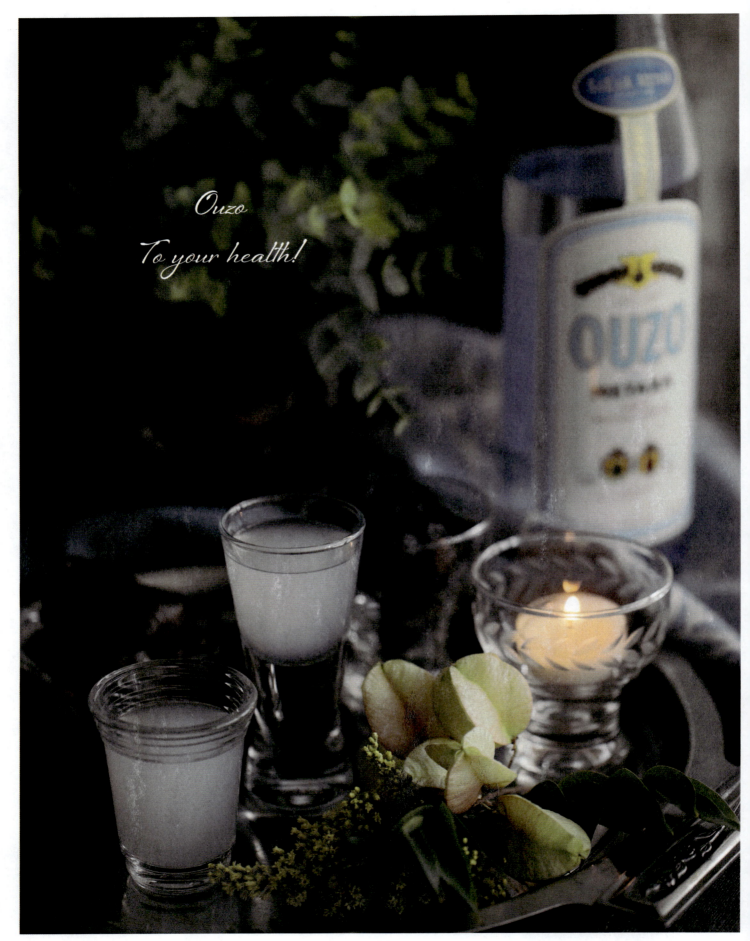

Ouzo
To your health!

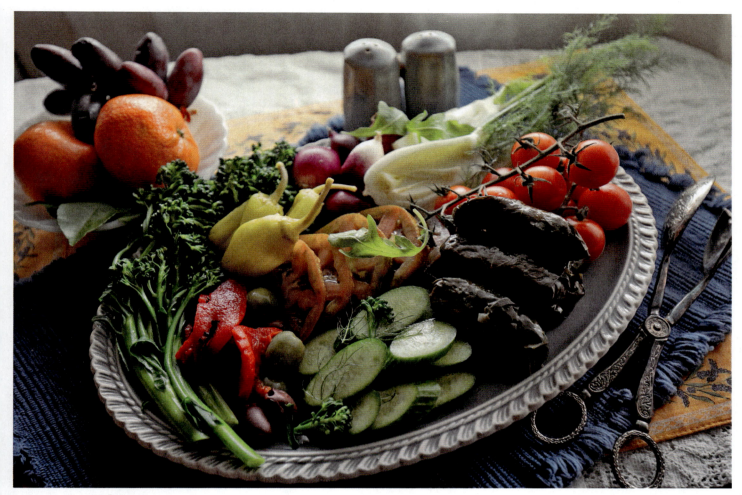

Veggie Platter

Makes 4 to 8 mezze portions.

Use whatever raw seasonal veggies that are available - add a few olives and a side of fruit like grapes or tangerines. I also like to keep a can of dolmades on hand, so I'm ready at any time to put together a simple, and substantial mezze platter. We like Tamek Stuffed Vine Leaves brand dolmades.

Ingredients

- Broccolini – blanched
- Cucumber slices
- Fennel
- Greek peppers
- Olives
- Radishes
- Red bell peppers raw or from a jar
- Tomatoes
- Or some of your favorite veggies

Directions

1. Wash veggies thoroughly and dry with paper towels.
2. Leave small veggies whole.
3. Slice large veggies like cucumbers and/or roasted peppers from a jar.
4. Place veggies on platter - serve with optional "Tzatziki Dressing" on page 33 or "Greek Salad Dressing" on page 31.

To blanch the broccolini:

Or other veggie like broccoli or green beans – bring a medium pot of salted water to a boil. Drop veggie into the boiling water and cook JUST until the veggie turns bright green – approximately 1 minute. Drain and submerge in a bowl with ice water until chilled through. Drain, pat dry, and place on platter.

Gyro Slider with Grilled Veggies

- I call these gyros "sliders" because they are small - made with mini-pitas or mini-naans (I prefer the naans - shh don't tell yia yia)
- For each slider: 1 mini pita or mini naan - grilled on both sides just until warm
- Your choice of grilled veggie(s)
- Chopped tomato, sliced onion, sliced cucumber.
- Top with Tzatziki or Tahini Dressing.

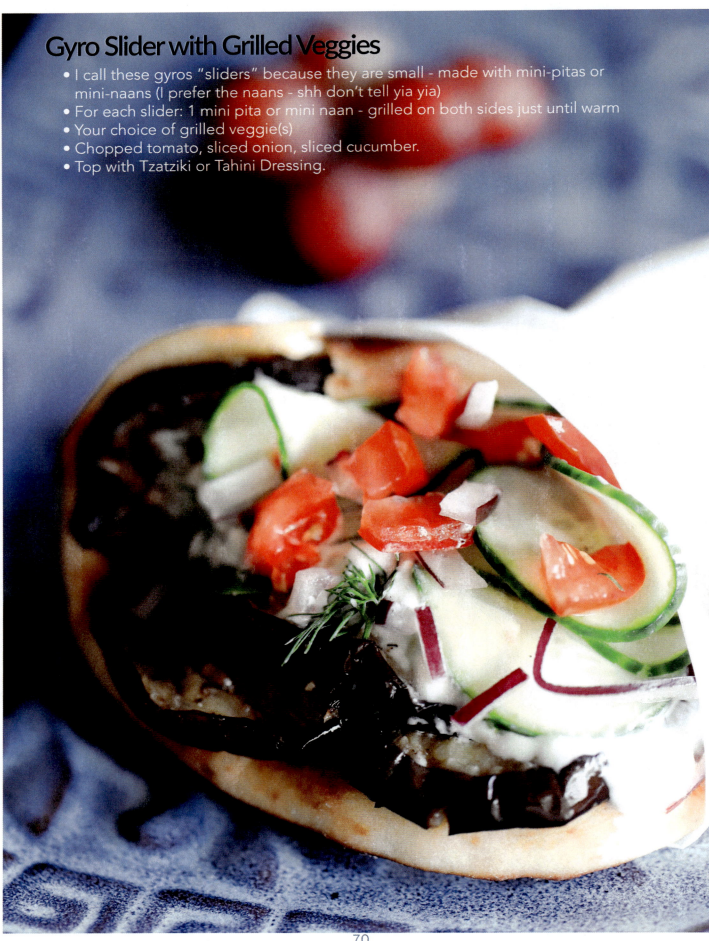

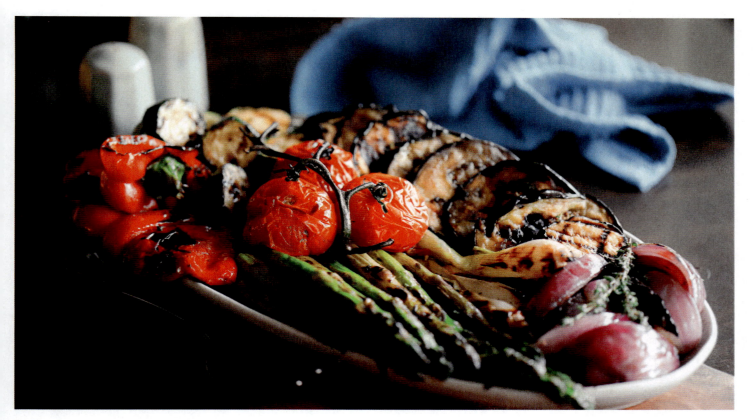

Grilled Veggie Platter

Grilling a big platter of colorful veggies makes a relaxing and casual mezze get-together. Grill whatever seasonal produce is available. Then gather round to share stories, while enjoying the rich smoky flavors that only grilling can offer.

Put out sides of hummus, "Schug" on page 148, "Gremolata" on page 142, and "Olive Tapenade" on page 55 with grilled pita or Greek bread. Add fruit, cold Mythos beer and "Iced Orange Tea with" on page 126 for refreshing touches of hospitality.

Ingredients

- Asparagus
- Eggplant
- Tomatoes
- Green Onions
- Peppers
- Red onions
- Zucchini
- Or your favorite seasonal veggies
- Olive oil
- Greek Seasoning Blend or dried oregano and dried mint
- Unrefined sea salt

Directions

1. Preheat grill to 400° F – 450° F
2. Try to slice veggies the about the same thickness – and not too thin so they don't fall between the grill grates.
3. Leave tomatoes & asparagus whole.
4. Place veggies in large bowl - drizzle with olive oil to coat, lightly salt, and lightly sprinkle with "Greek Seasoning Blend" on page 142 or sprinkle with a pinch dried oregano and dried mint.
5. Lay veggies on the hot grill crosswise so they don't fall through the grates.
6. Close the grill lid and cook for 5 minutes.
7. Open the grill, flip the veggies over and grill another few minutes.
8. Different veggies take different times to cook – so remove the veggie as they become cooked through.
9. Arrange on plate - serve at warm or at room temperature

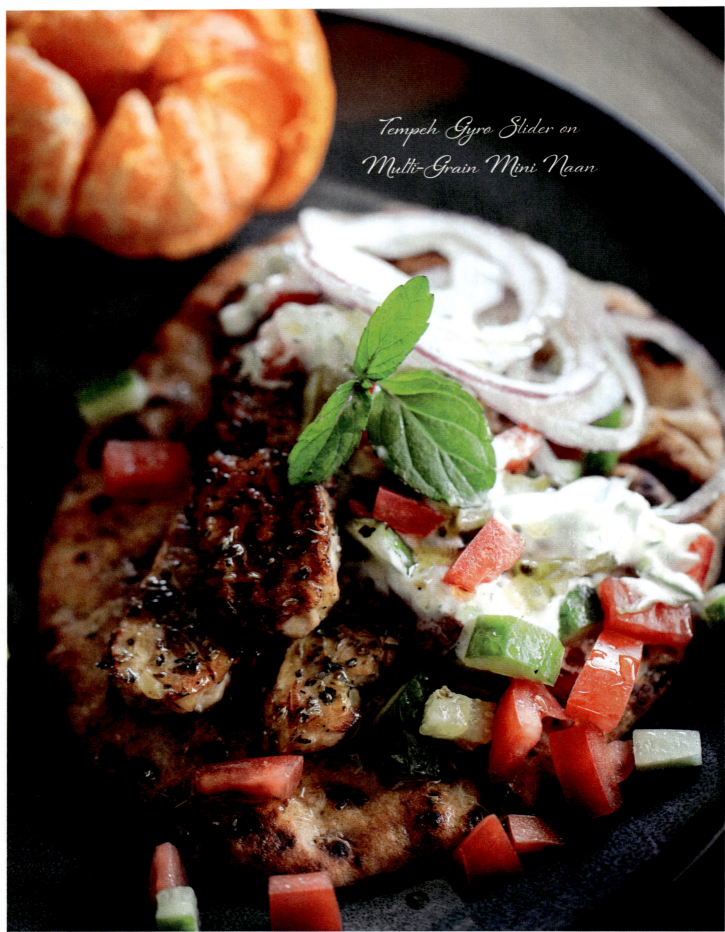

Tempeh Gyro Slider on Multi-Grain Mini Naan

Tempeh Gyro Slider

Makes 4 mezze-sized sliders.

Greeks and gyros are a thing. This plant-based gyro recipe is delicious enough for Zeus himself!

Ingredients

- 12-ounce package tempeh
- 1 small white onion grated
- 1-garlic clove mashed into a paste or through a press
- 1-tablespoon fresh lemon juice
- 1/2 teaspoon dried marjoram
- ½ teaspoon ground rosemary
- ½ teaspoon ground oregano
- ½ teaspoon ground black pepper
- ¼ teaspoon sea salt
- 1-tablespoon olive oil plus a little more to sauté the tempeh
- 1-teaspoon liquid smoke
- 4 Mini multigrain pita or ancient mini-naan
- 2 Roma or plum tomatoes diced
- 2 mini or Persian cucumber diced
- 1 small onion sliced
- Pinch of dried oregano
- Dress with Tzatziki, Tahini Dressing or vegan sour cream
- Extra light olive oil for shallow frying.

Tempeh Directions

1. Heat water in medium pot until boiling.
2. Cut tempeh in half – place in boiling water, reduce heat and simmer tempeh, covered for 15 minutes.
3. Remove from water - cool until warm
4. Cut into ¼ inch strips and place in Ziploc bag with marinade.

Marinade & Gyro Strips Directions

1. Place grated onion, garlic, lemon juice, marjoram, ground rosemary, ground oregano, black pepper, sea salt, tablespoon olive oil and smoke into Ziploc bag.
2. Press bag to blend mixture together.
3. Place tempeh strips into bag with marinade – turn bag several times to coat strips with marinade.
4. Marinate in fridge for 3 hours or overnight.
5. Heat large skillet on low heat.
6. Brush skillet with a little olive oil.
7. Remove strips from marinade and cook 3 to 4 minutes on each side or until golden brown
8. Brush tempeh with more olive oil and sprinkle with dried oregano.
9. Serve on small warmed pita bread, Ancient Grain Naan or collard leaf
10. Top with tomatoes, onions, cucumbers and "Tzatziki Dressing" on page 33 or "Tahini Dressing" on page 33.

Green Gyro

Make gyro as directed but omit the pita or naan, and serve on a small collard or kale leaf.

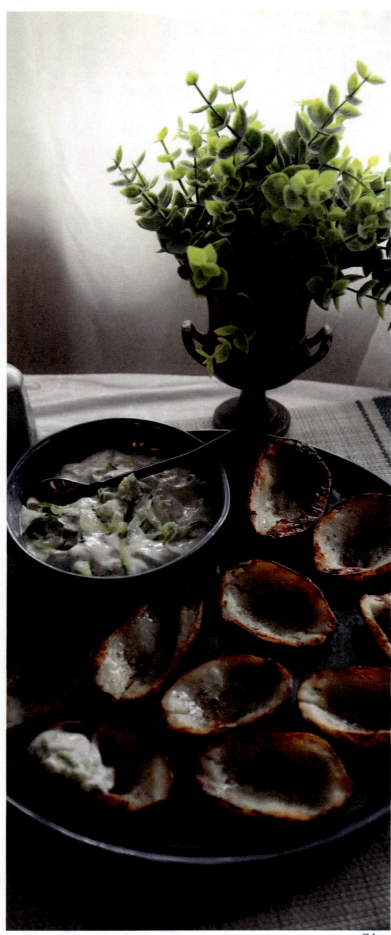

Potato Skins Greek Style with Lemon & Oregano

Makes 6 to 12 mezze servings.

Ingredients

- 1 pound organic baby or small potatoes – I used 6 small Idaho potatoes
- 2 tablespoons olive oil - divided
- 1 tablespoon lemon juice
- Unrefined sea salt
- Dried oregano

Directions

1. Preheat oven to 425°F
2. Scrub potatoes and dry with paper towels.
3. Arrange on parchment lined baking sheet.
4. Drizzle with 1 tablespoon olive oil and toss potatoes with your hands to coat.
5. Lightly sprinkle with unrefined sea salt on all sides.
6. Bake on center rack of preheated oven until tender, about 30 to 40 minutes.
7. Remove potatoes from oven and cool enough to handle.
8. Slice potatoes in half lengthwise.
9. Using a spoon, scoop out the white flesh - leave 1/8-inch layer inside the potato shell.
10. Reserve potato flesh for other use.
11. Increase oven temperature to 450°F.
12. Place potatoes hollowed side down, skin side up on baking sheet with parchment paper.
13. Bake in 450°F oven for 10 minutes.
14. Whisk 1 tablespoon olive oil with 1 tablespoon lemon juice.
15. Flip potatoes over, using pastry brush - brush the inside flesh with olive oil and lemon juice.
16. Sprinkle each with small amount of dried oregano.
17. Bake until crispy, 10 to 15 minutes.
18. Serve hot or warm with Tzatziki Sauce, crumbled plant-based feta, Olive Tapenade, Tabouli, or your favorite topping.

Greek Nachos

Makes 4 to 6 mezze portions.

Ingredients

- Pita chips
- ½ cup cooked lentils drained well
- 2 Persian cucumbers diced
- 12 Castelvetrano & Kalamata olives, coarsely chopped
- Tomatoes, chopped
- Purple onion, diced
- Jalapeno pepper thinly sliced
- Plant-based feta cheese
- "Schug" on page 148
- "Tzatziki Dressing" on page 33

Directions

1. Place pita on serving plate.
2. Spoon lentils on top of chips.
3. Top lentils evenly with cucumbers, olives, tomatoes, onion, and jalapeno.
4. Place bits of plant-based feta on top of veggies.
5. Dribble top with small dollops of Schug and Tzatziki.
6. Serve immediately.

For a quicker version, replace the lentils with hummus.

Crispy!

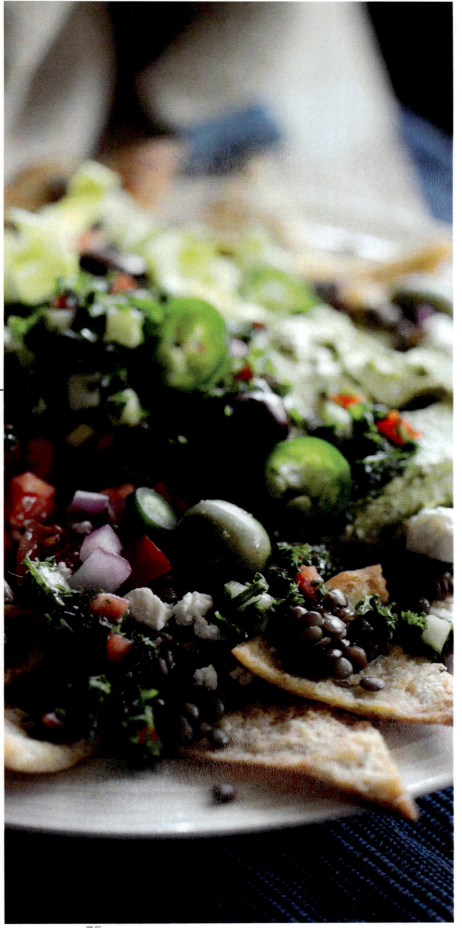

Keftedes

Makes 16 to 20 keftedes.

AIR FRIED KEFTEDES OR SHALLOW PAN FRIED

Keftedes were possibly my family's most coveted comfort food. Yia yia and my mother made the traditional herb-infused meatballs with ground beef or a combination of beef and lamb. They were a mouthwatering mezze that we looked forward to at every get-together. And so when reworking my favorites with plant-based versions, a recipe for keftedes was at the top of my list.

My mother served her keftedes with fresh lemon wedges. I serve my plant-based version with schug, which adds a punch of lemony freshness and a bolus of antioxidants.

Ingredients

- ½ cup chopped walnuts
- ½ cup old-fashioned oatmeal coarsely ground
- 1 cup cooked green or brown lentils drained
- ½ cup sweet onion grated
- ½ cup raw Idaho potato grated with peel
- 1 teaspoon dried parsley
- Lemon zest from 1 organic lemon
- 1-tablespoon fresh lemon juice
- 2 teaspoons dried mint
- 1 teaspoon dried oregano
- ¾ teaspoon unrefined sea salt
- 3 tablespoons chia seeds finely ground in coffee grinder
- 2 tablespoons vital wheat gluten
- Extra light olive oil to shallow fry or alternatively toss the keftedes with olive oil to coat and air fry.

Directions

1. Add walnuts and oatmeal to a food processor fitted with a steel blade. Pulse until coarsely ground – about 10 pulses.
2. Add cooked and drained lentils to the food processor with walnuts and oatmeal. Pulse to blend, approximately another 10 pulses.
3. Transfer mixture from food processor to a medium bowl.
4. Add the grated sweet onion, grated potato, lemon zest, lemon juice, dried mint, oregano, and salt – using hands, mix ingredients together.
5. Add chia seeds and gluten if using. Toss and knead with hands until mixture binds together to form a ball.
6. Set the mixture aside for 30 minutes for flavors to blend.
7. Using a small cookie scoop or a tablespoon, scoop up a heaping portion of mixture and roll between palms to make "meat" balls.

Air Fry

1. Drizzle a little olive oil onto keftedes – toss to coat on all sides.
2. Place in air fryer basket, and fry at 350°F for 12 minutes.
3. Serve at room temperature with lemon wedges and "Schug" on page 148 or if you prefer,"Tzatziki Dressing" on page 33.

Shallow Fry Keftedes on Stove-Top

1. In a medium frying pan, heat approximately ¼ inch of olive oil over medium low heat.
2. Shallow fry the keftedes in the oil 3 to 4 minutes on each side.
3. Drain on paper towels.

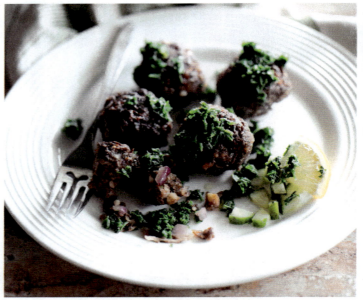

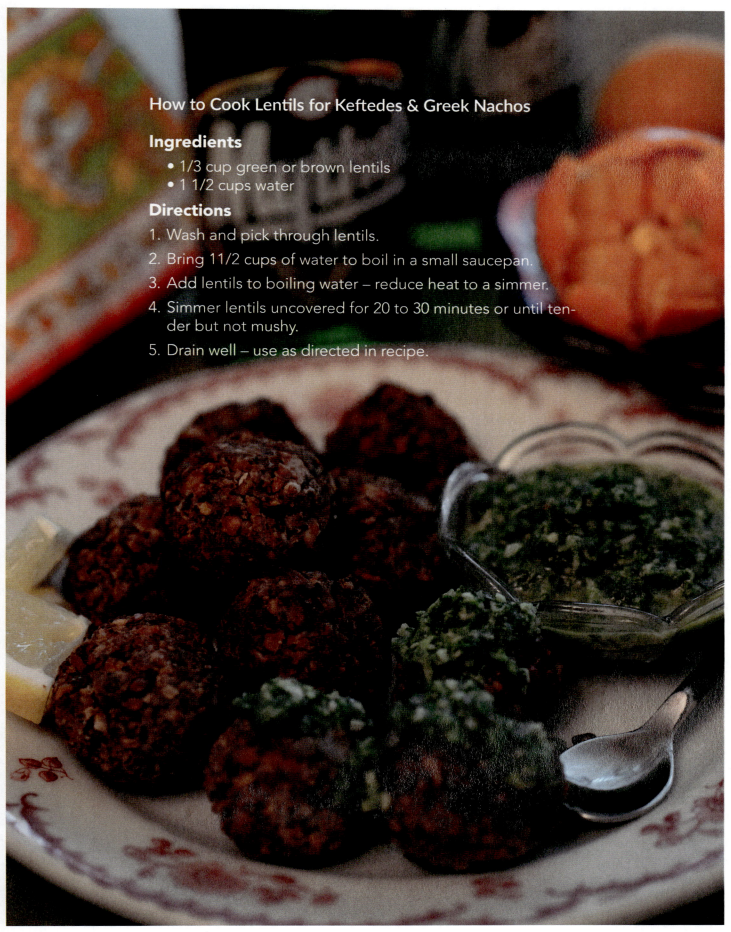

How to Cook Lentils for Keftedes & Greek Nachos

Ingredients
- 1/3 cup green or brown lentils
- 1 1/2 cups water

Directions
1. Wash and pick through lentils.
2. Bring 1 1/2 cups of water to boil in a small saucepan.
3. Add lentils to boiling water – reduce heat to a simmer.
4. Simmer lentils uncovered for 20 to 30 minutes or until tender but not mushy.
5. Drain well – use as directed in recipe.

Everyday Koliva

Koliva is much more than a simple recipe. Koliva is an ancient ritual "pie" served at Greek funeral receptions and memorial services. It's made with boiled wheat berries, dried fruits, nuts, honey, and spices. The person who prepares the koliva whispers prayers for the deceased throughout the cooking process. It's then decorated with a coating of confectioner's sugar, a cross-designed with fruits and nuts, and the departed's initials. The koliva receives additional blessings from the Greek priest before being served.

During my holistic nurse's training, I learned that all matter has energy. Energy creates memorable food experiences — some good and some bad. Koliva is made with earthly gifts steeped in prayers. The best way I can explain koliva's flavor is to say it's like a sweet taste of love, comfort, and joy. It's a memorial dish that was present at every Greek funeral reception I attended. Koliva holds so many meaningful memories for me that, as an adult, I miss it at non-Orthodox gatherings. This is why I wish to share this beautiful recipe - and the ancient love and prayer-energy it brings to the table.

Many eat koliva outside of traditional Orthodox settings. It's high in fiber, B vitamins, iron, and protein. Organic wheatberries are in their most whole and healthful form.

Koliva makes a delicious superfood breakfast with a little nondairy creamer or a healthy taste of sweet for dessert. It also makes for friendly conversation at potlucks, and picnics or as a unique gift to lift spirits at any mezze gathering.

Makes 4 to 8 servings.

Ingredients

- 1-cup hard red wheat berries cooked
- ½ cup dried cherries or cranberries coarsely chopped
- ½ cup golden raisins coarsely chopped
- Seeds from 1 pomegranate
- ¼ cup walnuts finely chopped
- 1-tablespoon sesame seeds
- 1-tablespoon agave
- 1-teaspoon cinnamon
- Optional confectioner's sugar

Directions

1. Wash wheat berries thoroughly.
2. Soak the berries in spring or filtered water for 4 hours or overnight.
3. Add berries to medium saucepan and cover with 3 inches of water.
4. Gently simmer the wheat berries on low heat in lightly salted water for about 45 minutes – the berries should be whole, plump and chewy – do not overcook or the berries will burst and become gummy.
5. Strain and rinse in cool water.
6. Place berries on clean kitchen towel, pat them dry – at this point you may put them in a Ziploc bag with paper towels and refrigerate before proceeding with the recipe.
7. Chop the dried cherries, raisins and walnuts into coarse, evenly sized pieces.
8. In medium bowl, combine the wheatberries with cherries, raisins, walnuts, pomegranate seeds, sesame seeds, cinnamon and agave.
9. Spoon the koliva into a pie dish or nice serving dish.
10. Optional: sprinkle confectioner's sugar over the top.
11. Store in refrigerator covered in the refrigerator.
12. Will keep for 4 to 5 days in fridge.

Note: I buy my wheatberries in bulk at local health food stores like Whole Foods. Bob's Red Mill also sells quality wheatberries.

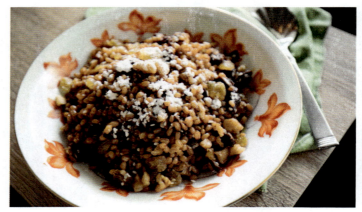

Horta - Greens

Horta is a Greek word for "weeds" and are the most popular greens eaten in Greece. We were told stories that our yia yia plucked fresh bunches of horta out of her back yard or from vacant lots on the island in the Aegean where she grew up. In Tarpon Springs, we purchased greens, usually dandelions, from the local market. My mother would wash them, drop them in a salty pot of boiling water then reduce the heat to simmer. She stewed them on low, it seemed, for 2 to 3 hours. They were silky, soft, and melt in your mouth. She doused them with olive oil and a spritz of fresh lemon juice. She used the leftover cooking liquid, that was vitamin and mineral-rich, to make soup.

Horta includes a variety of different greens. I find the best selection in Asian food markets. Some of the greens I use are dandelion greens, amaranth, and callaloo. A bag of Power Greens are a wonderful substitute for horta.

Ingredients

- 1 or 2 bunches of greens like dandelion thoroughly washed or a bag of pre-washed Power Greens
- Olive oil
- Fresh lemon wedges
- Salt to your desired taste

Directions

1. Thoroughly wash greens.
2. Fill large pot with filtered or spring water and a little salt.
3. Bring to a boil over high heat.
4. Add greens to boiling water, reduce heat, and simmer uncovered for 15 minutes or longer if you prefer your horta softer.
5. Drain and serve with lemon wedges, olive oil, and salt to your taste.
6. Serve them hot, warm or at room temperature.

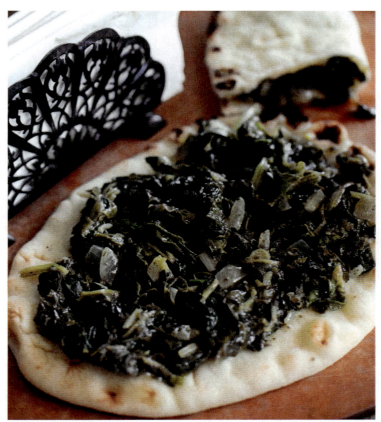

Horta Hand Pie

1. Fold a spoonful of drained, cooked greens in a warm min-pita or mini-naan.
2. Serve immediately.
3. Optional: in a small skillet, saute a small chopped onion in a little olive oil over medium heat for 3 to 5 minutes or until starting to brown. Toss with greens.

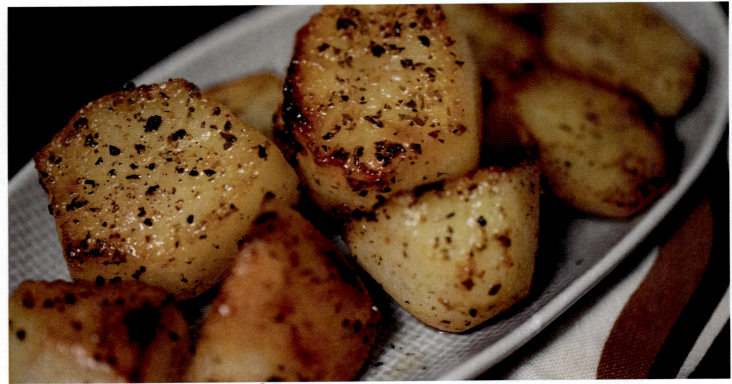

Lemony Greek Roasted Potatoes

Yield 4 to 8 servings

This is my family's favorite potato recipe. They are a little crusty on the outside, fluffy and creamy on the inside, and lemony throughout. It's true - Greek lemon potatoes are one of the secret ingredients for a happy life.

Ingredients

- 4 baking potatoes, peeled and cut into 1-inch rounds
- 1 cup water
- 1/3 cup lemon juice
- 1/3 cup olive oil
- 2 teaspoons dried oregano
- 1 teaspoon dried onion flakes
- Sea salt
- Fresh ground pepper

Directions

1. Preheat oven to 425°F.
2. Place potato rounds in glass baking dish together with water, lemon juice, olive oil, oregano, and dried onion.
3. Sprinkle with sea salt and a few grinds of black pepper.
4. Using hands, toss the potatoes to coat with the ingredients.
5. Bake uncovered, on center rack of 425°F preheated oven for 1 hour.
6. Turn potatoes and spoon some of the lemony sauce onto the potatoes several times while baking.
7. Add small amounts of water during baking if needed.
8. After an hour, potatoes should be lightly brown on edges and easily pierced with fork.

Persian Pizza

Ingredients for individual pizza

- 1 small pita, naan, or pide (Turkish oblong flatbread)
- 1 to 2 tablespoons hummus
- 1 tablespoon chopped and massaged kale
- 1/2 mini or Persian cucumber sliced into thin rounds
- 4 grape tomatoes cut into halves
- 3 oil cured or Moroccan olives, seeded and cut into halves
- Few thin slices of red onion
- 2 teaspoons olive oil
- 1 teaspoon fresh lemon juice
- 1/2 teaspoon hemp seeds
- Pinch dried oregano

Directions

1. Heat pita on grill or under broiler.
2. Quickly smear pita with hummus.
3. Top with cucumbers, tomatoes, olives, and red onion.
4. Drizzle with olive oil & lemon juice
5. Sprinkle with hemp seeds
6. Top with a pinch of dried oregano.
7. Serve immediately.

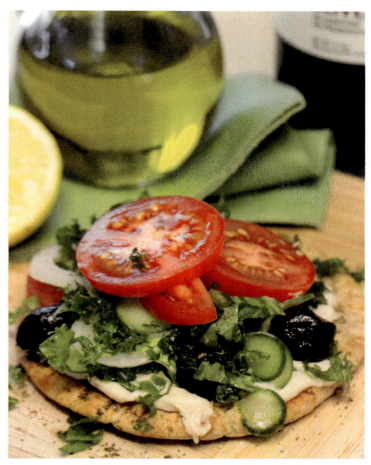

Persian Pizza on Mini Multigrain Naan

Persian Pizza on Turkish Pide

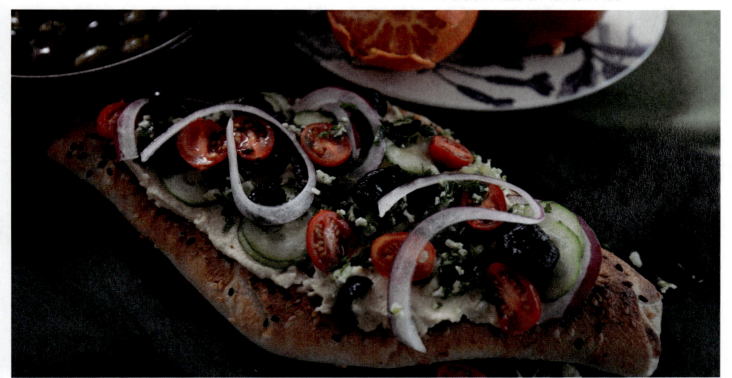

Power Greens in Phyllo

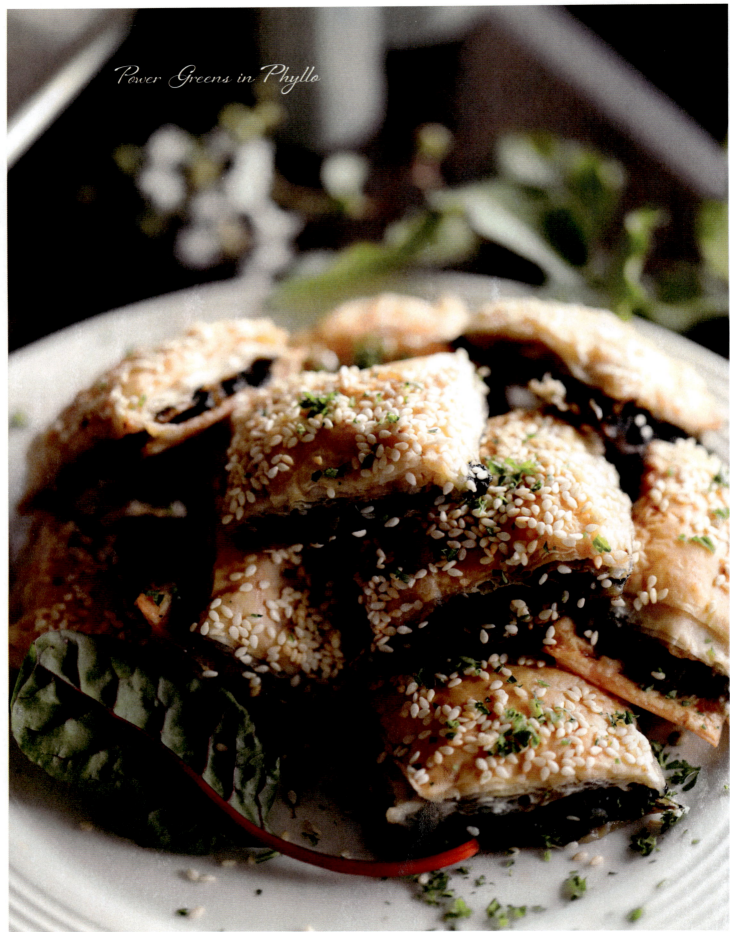

Power Greens in Phyllo recipe

Makes 16 to 24 mezze portions.

Greek spinach pie, spanakopita, is a favorite mezze. I make a superfood version by using power greens. In addition to spinach, a bag of power greens includes chard and kale. This gives the recipe a higher nutritional footprint.

I prepare my greens pie in free-form on a parchment lined baking sheet. This makes the slab easier to slice, quicker to cook, and it yields crispier squares.

Plan ahead. Phyllo is sold frozen. You can find it in the freezer section of the grocery store near puff pastry and frozen pie crusts. Phyllo works best thawed overnight in the refrigerator. Even better if thawed a in the fridge for a day or two before using.

Ingredients

- 1 tablespoon olive oil
- 1 sweet onion coarsely chopped
- 1 pound power greens
- 1 teaspoon dried dill
- 1 teaspoon dried mint
- 1 teaspoon dried sumac
- ½ teaspoon onion salt
- ½ pound, or approximately 24 sheets of phyllo dough
- ¼ cup plant-based butter
- ¼ cup olive oil
- 1 teaspoon fresh lemon juice
- 2 tablespoons sesame seeds

Directions

1. Preheat oven to 350° F.
2. Line a large baking sheet with parchment paper.
3. Heat large skillet over medium-low heat.
4. Add tablespoon of olive oil and onions to skillet – cook stirring until onions become translucent and start to turn brown - approximately 5 minutes.
5. Add power greens to the skillet with onions – toss and turn the greens until they wilt.
6. Stir in dill, mint, sumac, and onion salt.
7. Remove the skillet from the burner cool to room temperature – greens need to cool before spreading onto phyllo so it doesn't become gummy.
8. Drain excess liquid from the greens in a colander in the sink.
9. Place butter in small sauce pan and melt over low heat - stir ¼ cup of olive oil into melted butter.
10. Cover phyllo sheets with a damp kitchen towel.
11. Working quickly – lay a sheet of phyllo onto parchment lined baking sheet - using a pastry brush, lightly brush the sheet with the melted butter and olive oil mixture.
12. Lay a second layer on top of the first phyllo sheet – lightly brush with butter and olive oil mixture.
13. Repeat with 10 more layers for a total of 12 phyllo sheets for the bottom of your greens pie – lightly brushing each layer with melted butter and olive oil.
14. Evenly spoon the cooled and drained greens onto the phyllo sheets.
15. Lay a phyllo sheet on top of the greens layer, and brush with melted butter and olive oil mixture.
16. Repeat with the remaining phyllo – you should have approximately 12 sheets total for the top layers.
17. Using your hands, gently press the top layer of phyllo onto the other layers and greens.
18. Sprinkle the top of the rectangle evenly with sesame seeds.
19. Using a pizza wheel or sharp knife, cut into squares – you should have 16 to 24 squares depending on your desired size - try to leave slight spaces between squares.
20. Bake on the center rack of a preheated 350°F oven for 30 to 35 minutes or until golden brown.
21. Serve warm or at room temperature.
22. Store cooled leftover squares in a Ziploc bag in the fridge for 2 to 3 days.
23. Rewarm – re-crisp in a 350°F oven for 10 to 15 minutes.

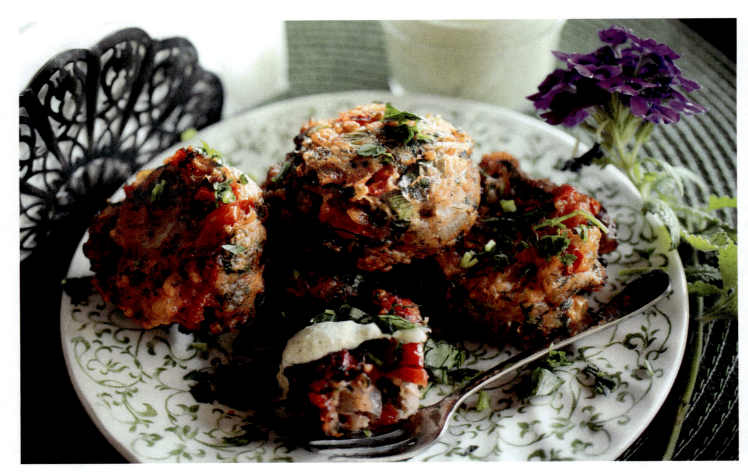

Tomato Keftedes

Makes 10 to 12 keftedes.

Ingredients

- 2 cups seeded tomatoes, diced
- 1 small onion, finely chopped
- 5 green onions (white and green parts) finely sliced
- 1 small bunch curly parsley chopped
- 1-teaspoon dried dill
- 1 teaspoon dried mint
- 2 teaspoons dried oregano
- 1 cup unbleached all purpose flour
- 1-teaspoon baking powder
- ½ teaspoon sea salt
- Extra light olive oil for frying
- Tahini Dressing

Directions

1. In a large bowl, combine the tomatoes, onion, green onions, parsley, dill, mint, oregano, flour, baking powder and salt
2. Mix well with a spoon or hands until combined.
3. Taste and add more salt and pepper if desired.
4. Allow to sit for 15 minutes so flour can absorb veggie liquids
5. Heat approximately ½ inch of oil in a frying pan over medium heat
6. Carefully drop heaping tablespoons of batter at a time in the oil and fry until golden brown flipping carefully to prevent the fritters from falling apart
7. Drain Tomato Keftedes on paper towels to absorb excess oil.
8. Serve immediately with "Tahini Dressing" on page 33 or vegan mayonnaise.

Stuffed Celery & Other Veggies

For a quick plate of mezzes stuff veggies that you may have on hand with hummus. Garnish with chopped tomatoes, olives, sprouts or microgreens.

Ingredients

- Celery ribs
- Cucumber
- Grape or cherry tomatoes
- "Hummus" on page 35
- Kalamata olives finely chopped
- Tomatoes finely chopped
- Sprouts or microgreens

Directions

1. Cut celery into 1-inch lengths
2. Slice hothouse cucumbers into rounds
3. Slice grape or cherry tomatoes in half.
4. Stuff or top with a little hummus.
5. Garnish with finely chopped olives, tomatoes, and sprinkle with sprouts or microgreens.

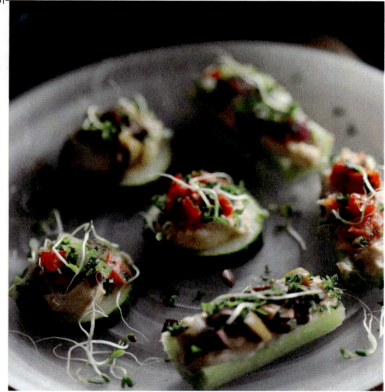

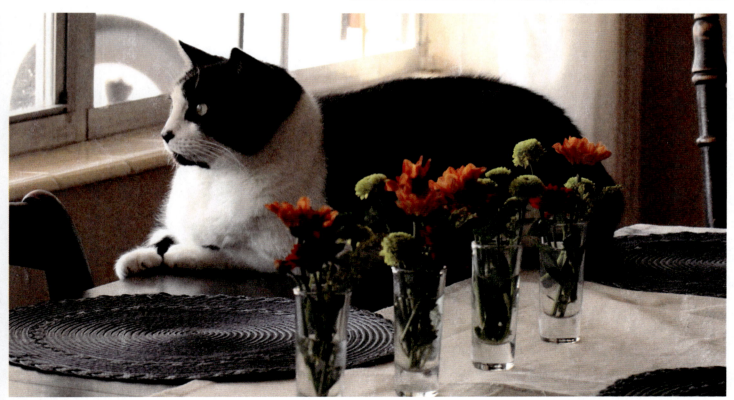

When time permits, make individual bouquets for my guests. I use an inexpensive bunch of flowers from the grocery store. I separate them into equal bouquets and place them in liqueur glasses that I picked up from a thrift store. (FYI - Romeo IS NOT allowed on the table!)

White Beans on Grilled Greek Toast

Makes 4 mezze servings.

The friars I cooked for were mostly Italian - and they loved big, white creamy cannellini beans. For a quick appetizer or light meal, I would make garlicky cannellini beans with tomatoes served over grilled toast. It became a plant-based favorite.

I make them by gently simmering canned cannellini beans with a little olive oil, grated onion, and minced garlic. I toss in a few grape tomatoes and cook just long enough to heat them through. Just before serving, I garnish with chopped fresh parsley and a few grinds of fresh pepper.

Grilling slices of Greek bread only takes a few minutes and enhances the flavor.

Ingredients

- 4 slices "Grilled Greek Toasts" on page 143 (or use Italian, French or other bread of choice)
- 2 tablespoons extra virgin olive oil
- ½ cup grated white onion
- 3 garlic clove, minced
- 15-ounce can of cannellini beans, drained and rinsed
- 1-½ cups filtered or spring water
- 8 grape tomatoes sliced in half
- Salt & pepper to your desired taste
- Serve with "Schug" on page 148 or "Gremolata" on page 142

Direction

1. Lightly brush Greek bread slices with olive oil (optional) or grill without oil
2. Grill slices on both sides on outside or stove-top grill
3. Heat 2 tablespoons of olive oil over medium low heat
4. Stir grated onions into olive oil – cook and stir until onions become soft and translucent – about 3 minutes
5. Stir in garlic, cook and stir another minute
6. Add beans, seasoning and water to skillet – simmer uncovered for 15 minutes
7. Stir in tomatoes and cook another minute or so to heat through.
8. Serve immediately on Grilled Greek Toasts with a topping of spicy Schug, Gremolata, & a scant drizzle of olive oil.

A Friars' Favorite!

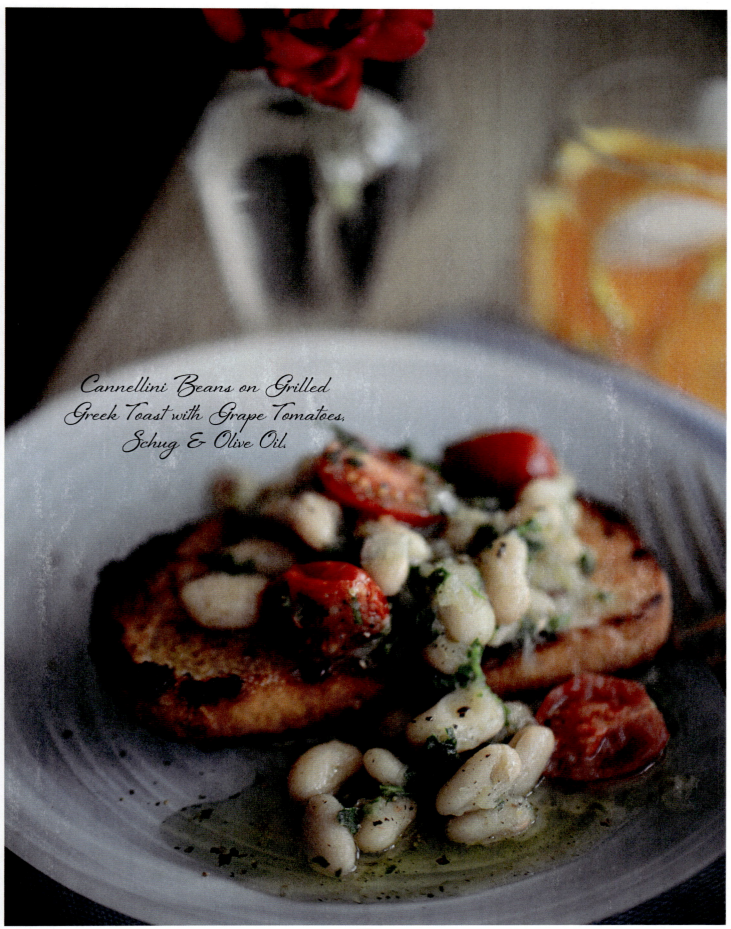

Cannellini Beans on Grilled Greek Toast with Grape Tomatoes, Schug & Olive Oil.

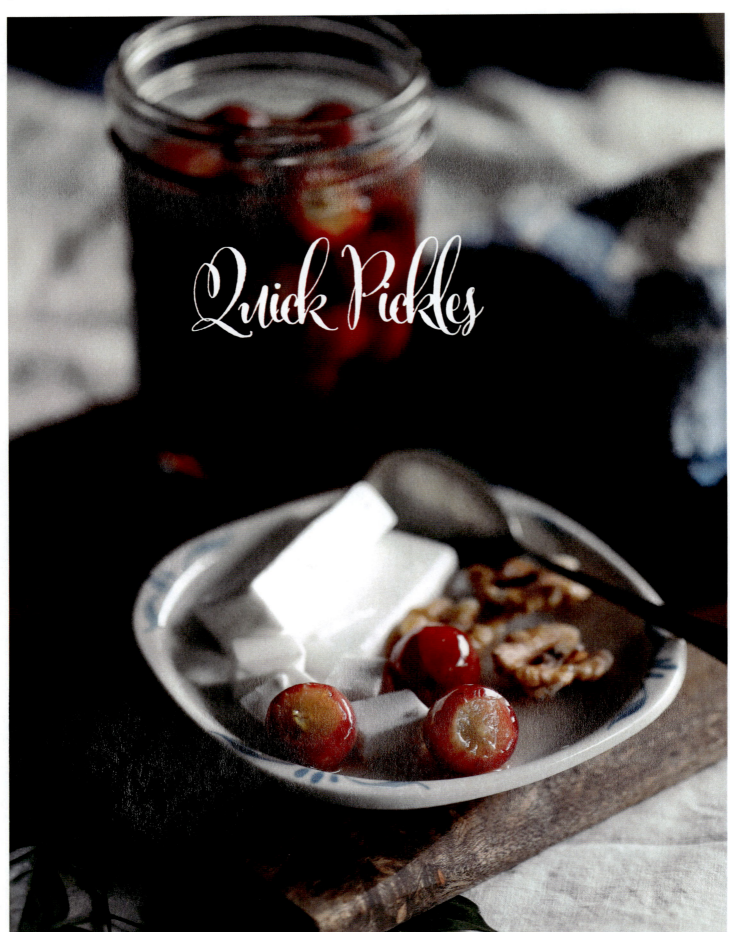

Pickled Grapes

Makes 1 pint jar.

These grapes are crisp, sweet, tart, and delicious all on their own. But when plant-based feta is served in the tangy, syrupy pickling brine – your taste buds will say, "Oh my yum."

Ingredients

- Red grapes to fill a pint jar – a little less than a pound
- ½ cup apple cider vinegar with mother
- 2 tablespoons water
- ½ cup raw cane sugar
- 1 cinnamon stick
- 2 whole cloves

Directions Pickled Grapes

1. Thoroughly wash the grapes, remove stems and cut a thin slice off of the stem end to allow the pickling syrup to infuse the grapes.
2. Fill a pint jar with grapes.
3. In a small saucepan, combine the vinegar, water, cane sugar, cinnamon, and cloves bring to a boil over medium heat.
4. Reduce heat to low and simmer for 5 minutes.
5. Pour hot vinegar solution with spices over the grapes.
6. Cover the jar with a lid and cool to room temperature.
7. Best if refrigerated overnight and severed chilled.
8. Store in the refrigerator – best if eaten within a week.
9. Optional: Serve with plant-based feta and nuts.

Pickled Red Onions

Makes 1 pint jar.

Crisp and tangy with a hint of sweet. These pickled onions add a pop of color to any mezze table – and a dimension of care and flavor to gyros, falafels, burgers, salads, and more. You can also whisk their brine into salad dressings.

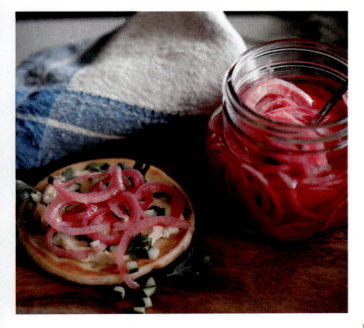

Ingredients Pickled onions

- I medium red onion, thinly sliced
- ½ cup water
- ½ cup apple cider vinegar with mother
- 1 tablespoon agave or maple syrup
- ½ teaspoon unrefined sea salt

Directions

1. Pack the onions into a clean pint glass jar.
2. Place the water, vinegar, agave, and sea salt in to a small sauce pan and bring to a boil over medium heat.
3. Pour the hot vinegar mixture over the onions in the jar.
4. Use a knife inserted down into the jar to release any air bubbles.
5. Cover and cool the onions to room temperature.
6. Store covered in refrigerator.
7. Serve as a condiment with mezzes.
8. Onions will keep for 2 weeks.

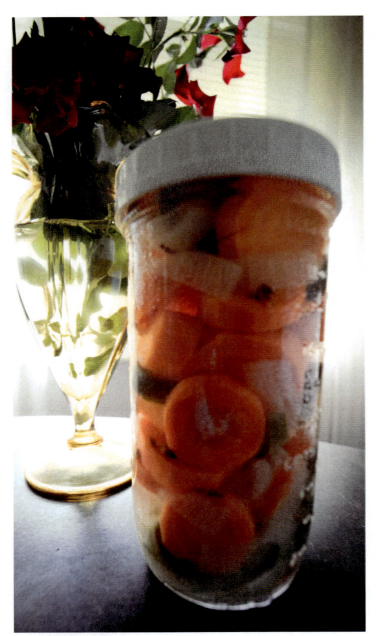

Pickled Carrots

Makes 1 1/2 pint jar.

I love to add pickled carrots to my mezze collection because of their bright orange energy and delicious earthy flavor.

Ingredients

- 1-cup apple cider vinegar
- 3/4-cup water
- 1 bay leaf
- 1-teaspoon oregano
- 1/2 teaspoon unrefined sea salt
- 1/2 large white onion, peeled and cut into ¼ inch slices
- 1 jalapeno sliced into ¼-inch rounds, seeds removed
- 2 carrots scrubbed, peeled and sliced into ½ inch discs

Directions

1. In a non-aluminum saucepan, heat vinegar, water, bay leaf, oregano and salt until boiling.
2. Turn off heat - add onion, carrot slices and jalapeno to hot liquid, put a lid on pot and bring to room temperature.
3. The hot liquid brine will pickle the veggies as they cool.
4. To serve, drain vegetables and offer as a compliment to other delicious mezzes.

Pickled Prunes

Note: while pickled prunes are simply amazing on their own — one of my very favorite ways to serve them, and their spiced liqueur, is in a fresh fruit salad.

Ingredients

- 1 lb. package pitted prunes
- 1 cinnamon stick
- 1-teaspoon whole cloves
- 1-teaspoon whole allspice
- 1-½ cups light brown sugar
- ¾ cups apple cider vinegar
- 2 cups water

Directions Pickled Prunes

1. Add all ingredients to saucepan.
2. Bring to a boil over medium heat, reduce heat and simmer uncovered for 30 minutes or until prunes are plump.
3. Serve warm or cold.

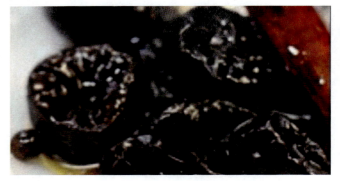

Pickled Turnips

Makes a 1 1/2 pint jar.

Ingredients

- 1-cup apple cider vinegar
- ½ cup filtered or bottled water
- 2 teaspoons sea salt
- 1 garlic clove thinly sliced
- 1 small beet – thoroughly washed, peeled, and cut into thin strips
- 2 small turnips – thoroughly washed, peeled, and cut into ½ inch strips
- 1 pint mason jars with a plastic lid

Directions

1. In small saucepan make brine by bringing vinegar, water salt and garlic slices to a boil.
2. Remove from heat.
3. Evenly distribute and pack beet and turnip strips into jars.
4. Pour vinegar into jar - fill jar to completely cover turnips – discard any leftover brine.
5. Cover with lid and refrigerate
6. Pickles will be good the next day and even better in 3 days – pickles will keep in refrigerator 2 to 3 weeks.
7. Serve on falafel sandwiches or as a beautiful side on your mezze table.

Earthy

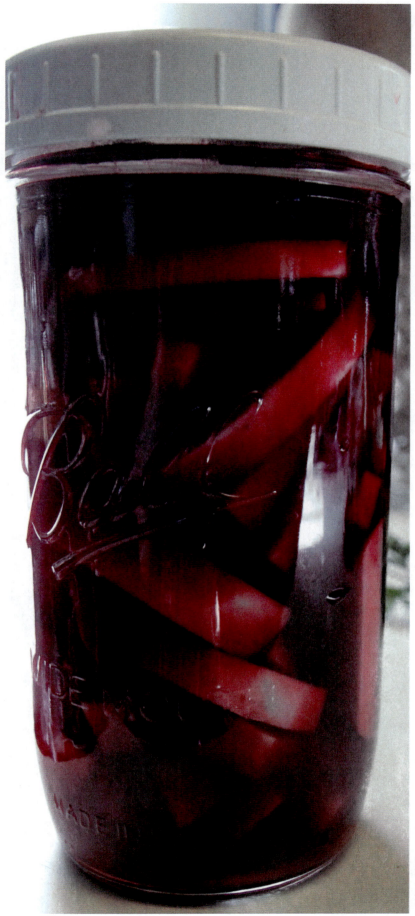

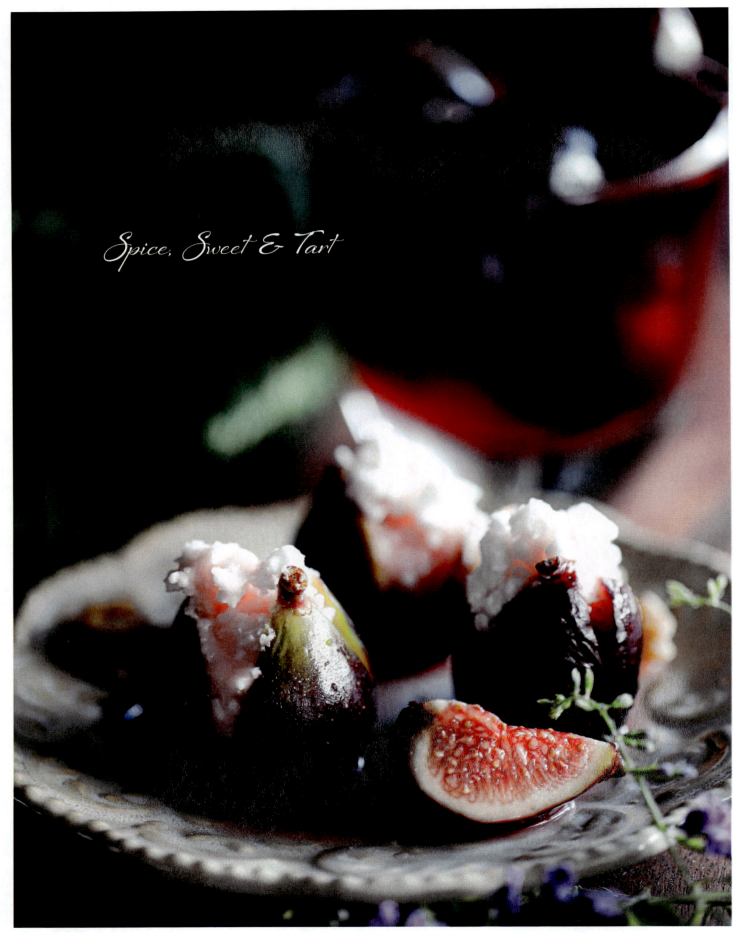

Spice, Sweet & Tart

Sweet Spiced Pickled Figs Stuffed with Feta

Makes 1 pint - approximately 10-12 figs.

The fig tree ripens its figs, and the vines are in blossom; they give forth fragrance. Arise, my love, my beautiful one, and come away.

Song of Songs 2:13

This recipe has it all - sweet, spice, tart, luscious, and beautiful.

Ingredients

- Fresh figs to almost fill a pint jar
- ½ cup apple cider vinegar with mother
- 2 tablespoons water
- ½ cup raw cane sugar
- 1 cinnamon stick
- 2 whole cloves
- 1 to 2 tablespoons plant-based feta - I like VioLife brand.

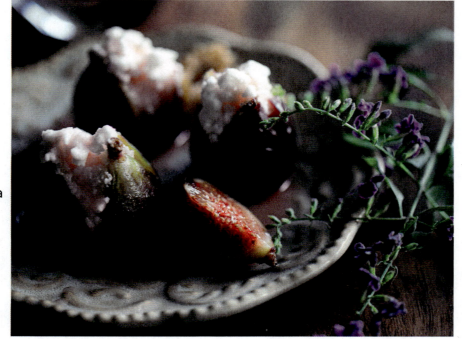

Directions

1. Thoroughly wash the figs and gently pat them dry with a paper towel.
2. With a sharp paring knife, cut an X into the top of each fig cutting half way through.
3. Place the amount of figs it takes to almost fill a clean pint glass jar – my fig count was 10.
4. In a small saucepan, combine the vinegar, water, cane sugar, cinnamon, and cloves bring to a boil over medium heat.
5. Reduce heat to low and simmer for 5 minutes.
6. Pour hot vinegar solution with spices over the grapes.
7. Cover the jar with a lid and cool to room temperature – turn the jar every few minutes during the cooling process to help the figs absorb the pickling liquid.
8. Once the figs come to room temperature they can be stuffed and served.
9. Store in the refrigerator – best if eaten within 4 days.
10. To Stuff - use a fork to mash 1 to 2 tablespoons of the feta until softened and fluffy.
11. Gently pull the fig quarters open.
12. Stuff each with ½ to 1 teaspoon of the fluffy feta cheese.
13. Spoon some of the sweet pickling brine over the tops of the figs.
14. Enjoy the figs around the mezze table.

Pickled Beets

My mother loved pickled beets. She frequently served them on Greek salad. I thought they were awful. I believed their earthiness contaminated any food they touched so I would carefully oust them from my plate. But times and my tastes have evolved. I have come to appreciate them and like my mom, I even have an affection for this dark purple root.

They are simple to prepare and I pretty much have a jar of beets in my fridge at all times. I serve them as a quick side or simply for a big-flavored snack. And it gives me a buzz to report that my grandchildren love them!

We're also hooked on any leftover pickled beet infused brine. We enjoy the vinegary liqueur in small amounts - sipped from a shot glass. My brother swears that pickled beets help to keep his blood pressure in normal range.

Ingredients

- 2 medium beets
- 1 cup apple cider vinegar
- 2 tablespoons agave – or more to your taste
- ¼ teaspoon ground cinnamon
- Pinch of ground cloves

Directions

1. Trim beets but do not peel or cut into the beet or a lot of the color will cook out.
2. Thoroughly wash beets.
3. Put them into a medium pot and cover with 3-4 inches of water.
4. Bring to a boil over medium-high heat, reduce heat to low and cook with lid slightly ajar until tender, about 1 hour.
5. Remove pot from stove and cool beets in pot until cool enough to handle.
6. Drain and cut the stem and root ends off of the beets.
7. Gently rub beets with paper towels – skin should slip off – or use a paring knife to remove the peel.
8. Cut beets in half and cut halves into quarters.
9. Add vinegar and agave to a clean, pint sized mason jar – cover with lid and shake to blend.
10. Add sliced beets to jar with vinegar and agave.
11. Store in refrigerator – will keep 2 weeks or longer.
12. Optional: just before serving, top with chopped cilantro.

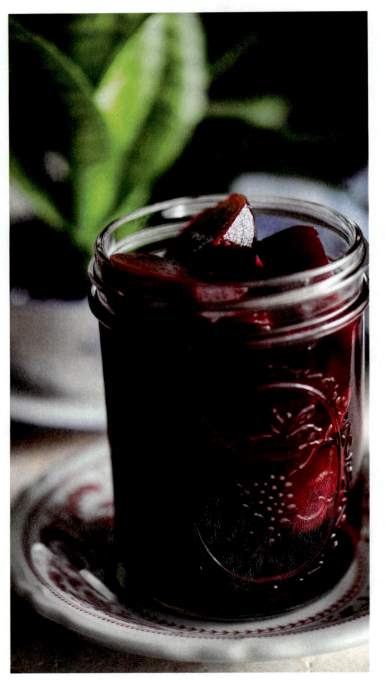

Sweets

Apple Slices with Agave & Cinnamon

• Possibly the easiest sweet mezze ever. Slices of your favorite apples, brushed with lemon juice, drizzled with agave, and dusted with cinnamon.

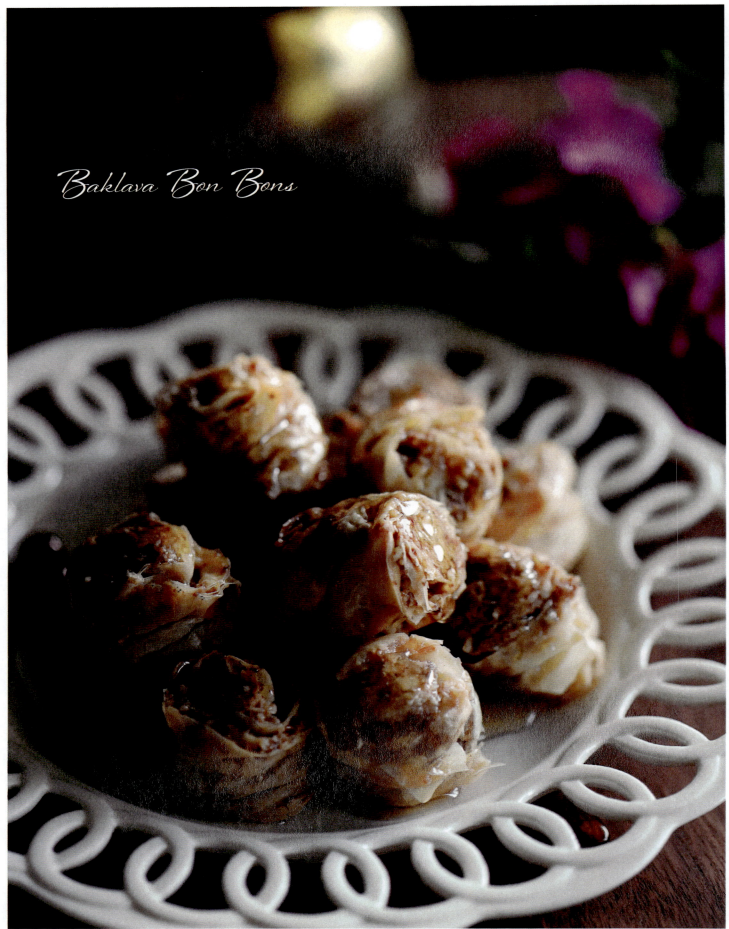
Baklava Bon Bons

Baklava Bon Bons

Saragli

Makes approximately 28 baklava bites to nibble.

Ingredients

- Make "Spiced Wine Syrup" on page 144, first
- 14 sheets of phyllo dough thawed overnight in the fridge
- ¼ cup plant-based butter
- ¼ cup olive oil
- 1 ¼ cups walnuts
- 2 teaspoons Spiced Wine Syrup
- ¾ teaspoon ground cinnamon
- Pinch of ground cloves
- Pinch of unrefined sea salt

Directions

1. Preheat oven to 325°F
2. Line a baking sheet with parchment paper.
3. Pulse the walnuts in a food processor together with 1 tablespoon Spiced Wine Syrup, cinnamon, cloves, and a pinch of salt.
4. Pulse until the mixture is blended and the walnuts are finely chopped.
5. Melt plant-based butter in a small saucepan over low heat until melted –
6. Stir olive oil into butter and remove from heat.
7. To prevent the phyllo from drying out – work quickly, and keep the phyllo covered with a clean damp kitchen towel.
8. Lay 1 sheet of phyllo dough on your work surface.
9. Using a pastry brush, lightly brush the phyllo with a little of the butter/oil mixture.
10. Cover the first with a second sheet of phyllo and brush with butter.
11. Evenly sprinkle 2 tablespoon of the walnuts onto the buttered phyllo.
12. Starting from short end, roll the phyllo dough into a cigar shape – not too tight.
13. Cut each roll into 1-inch pieces.
14. Place on parchment lined baking sheets, cut side up and gently press to slightly flatten.
15. Repeat the process until you run out of nuts and phyllo.
16. Lightly brush all nibbles with a little remaining butter.
17. Bake on the center rack of 325° F preheated oven for 20 to 25 minutes or until golden brown.
18. Remove the baklava nibbles from the oven and spoon the cooled syrup over the cookies.
19. Allow to sit until the cookies are thoroughly cooled.
20. Serve at room temperature.
21. Store cooled cookies in air tight container at room temperature. Will keep a couple of days.

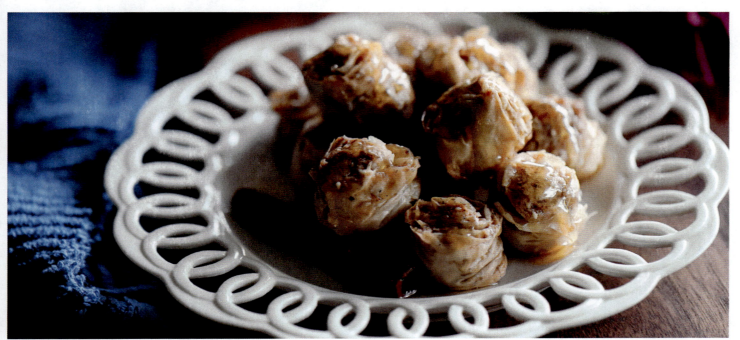

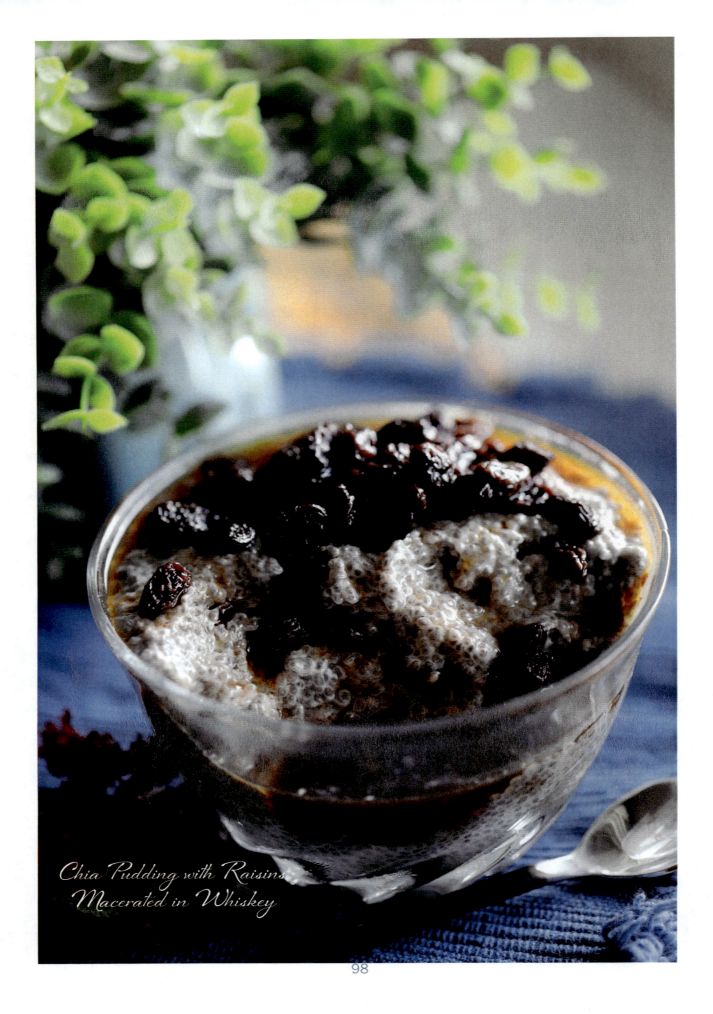
Chia Pudding with Raisins Macerated in Whiskey

Chia Pudding with Whiskey Macerated Raisins

Makes 6 to 8 small mezze portions.

Note: the whiskey in this recipe may not be suitable for the faint of heart.

Plan ahead. The raisins take at least 2 hours of soaking to become soft and deliciously plumped-up with whiskey.

My yia yia and mother didn't drink alcohol, but they always had booze in the house they used for cooking. Actually, we found yia yia laid out on the kitchen floor one afternoon. When my father aroused her, she said she was "all right, just a 'leedle' tired." Wonder if whiskey was involved? Anyway, she always had raisins, dried fruits, and/or nuts macerating in sherry, brandy, or whiskey. Boozy raisins gave her rice pudding it's signature tastiness.

I created this celestial chia pudding with the amazing flavors and lush mouth-feel of my yia yia's rice pudding. Even though this recipe is on the rich side, the chia seeds are loaded with antioxidants, quality protein, and omega 3; and it only takes a couple of spoonfuls to satisfy. I make it with homemade almond coconut milk creamer that's buttery with plant-fat but has zero cholesterol. There are no eggs or dairy. Then, I add raisins soaked in whiskey (Ballentine whiskey is plant-based and vegan friendly) and hot tea to make this pudding amazing!

Ingredients

- 2 cups homemade "Almond Coconut Cream" on page 132 – or your favorite nondairy creamer or milk
- 2 tablespoons maple syrup
- 1 teaspoon pure vanilla extract
- Pinch of salt
- ¾ cup chia seeds
- ½ cup raisins soaked in 1 tablespoon whiskey stirred with ¼ cup hot strong black tea for 2 to 3 hours or best if overnight
- Optional: coconut milk whipped cream or store bought nondairy whip cream & a sprinkle of cinnamon

Directions

1. In a small bowl, whisk together the almond coconut creamer, maple syrup, vanilla, and pinch of salt. Stir in the chia seeds.
2. Spoon half of the raisins with a little of the soaking liquid into the pudding.
3. The pudding will thicken in about 30 minutes – stir every 10 to 15 minutes.
4. Just before serving, spoon remaining raisins on top.
5. The pudding can be served immediately after it stiffens or chilled.
6. Store covered in refrigerator for up to 5 days.
7. Serve chilled with optional nondairy whipped cream & a sprinkle of cinnamon.
8. This recipe can be made a day or two ahead for a mezze gathering – the raisins only get better with time.

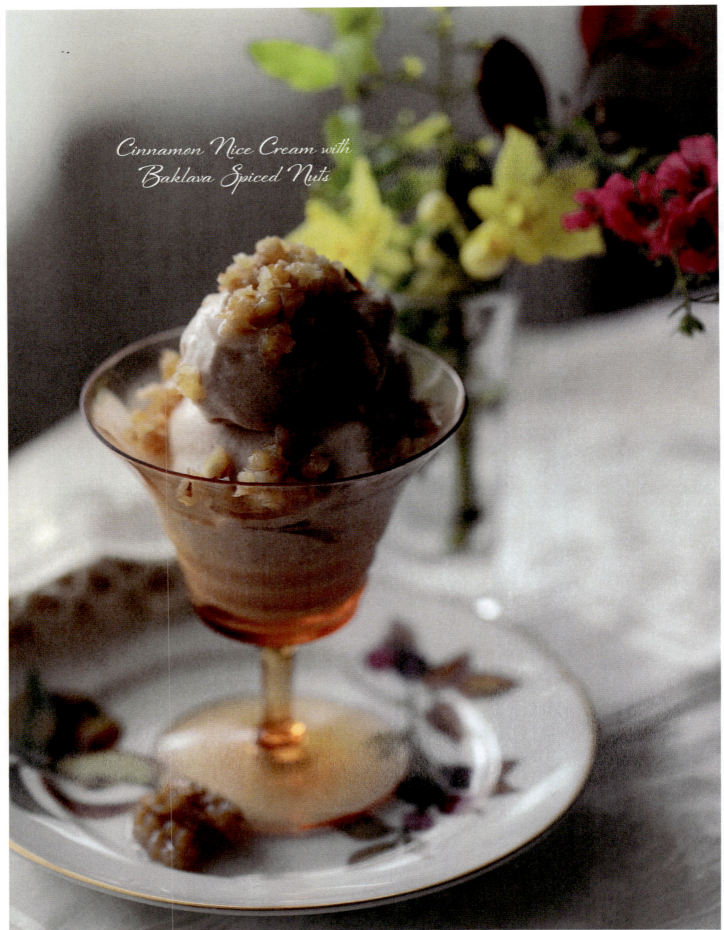

Cinnamon Nice Cream with Baklava Spiced Nuts

Cinnamon Nice Cream with Baklava Spiced Nuts

Makes 1 quart of Nice Cream.

I made this recipe for one of my plant-based cooking classes at a local health food store. I topped it with my baklava nut filling. The store manager took one bite, closed his eyes, and moaned, "that's the best thing I've ever tasted".

I'm not gonna lie - this recipe is time consuming . It's a tedious labor of love. But if you're looking for a plant-based dessert with a delicious taste of Greece, this is it!

Ingredients

- 1 cup cashews soaked overnight
- 1/2 cup young Thai coconut meat
- 1/2 cup agave
- 1 1/4 cups coconut water from the Thai coconut or nondairy milk
- 1/4 cup coconut oil melted
- 1 tablespoon vanilla extract (yes…that's right, a whole tablespoon)
- 1 teaspoon ground cinnamon
- Pinch of unrefined sea salt
- Optional: Baklava Spiced Nuts

Directions

Soak cashews in water in refrigerator overnight.

1. Drain cashews thoroughly and rinse.
2. Blitz cashews and other ingredients in blender until smooth – 1 to 2 minutes on high.
3. Freeze mixture in ice cream freezer according to manufacturer's instructions.
4. I like to blend the ice cream ingredients the morning of or day before I'm going to serve it and chill it in the fridge. Then a couple of hours before mezze guests arrive, I process it in the ice cream maker and store it in the freezer. IF you have leftovers, it will keep for a couple of weeks in the freezer but it becomes hard. Remove it from the freezer 15 to 20 minutes before serving for a softer texture.

Baklava Spiced Nuts

Ingredients

- 1/2 cup walnuts
- 1 teaspoon agave
- 1/4 teaspoon ground cinnamon
- Pinch of cloves
- Tiny pinch unrefined sea salt

Directions

1. Pulse ingredients together in small food processor until fine crumbs form.
2. Sprinkle on ice cream.

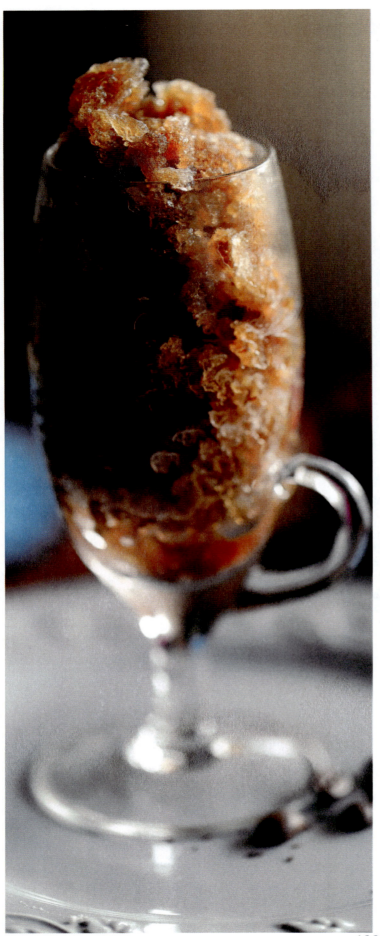

Greek Coffee Granita with Cardamom

Yields 6 mezze servings.

Ingredients

- 1 ½ cups "Greek Coffee" on page 123 strained, or strong American coffee
- 1 ½ tablespoons raw evaporated cane sugar or to your desired taste of sweet
- Pinch of ground cardamom

Directions

1. Make Greek coffee as directed - stir in a pinch of cardamom along with the sugar to hot coffee - you may need to make 3 or 4 pots of coffee depending on the size of your briki (Greek coffee pot) or simply use American coffee.
2. Strain coffee into a small, flat, freezer safe container – like a 2-inch deep casserole dish,- cool to room temperature then freeze.
3. Pour into a baking dish about ½ inch deep and place in freezer uncovered
4. Freeze until coffee just begins to freeze, about 45 minutes.
5. Coffee will begin to freeze from the edges but center will still be slushy.
6. Using a fork, stir the crystals from the edge of the granita into the center.
7. Chill in freezer until granita is almost frozen.
8. Stir, scrape, and break up clumps with fork about every 30 minutes for 2 hours or until it becomes light and fluffy.
9. You can serve it immediately or wrap with plastic wrap.
10. Best if eaten within a week – fluff with fork just before serving.

Fig & Anise Energy Bites

Makes 12 delicious mezze bites.

I have an intense affection for sweets; these fig bites are a healthy way to satisfy my craving. This is a modern recipe - updated with superfoods then combined with flavors common to a Greek kitchen. They make a perfect nosh for breakfast, a nutritious nibble for snacking, or as a lunchbox treat. I like to have them on hand to welcome pop-in family and friends. They make a perfect little something to go with a cup of coffee or tea.

I wanted this recipe to be simple – and so I tested it without toasting the oats and spices. But to me, the 10 minutes extra it takes to toast the oats with the spices is worth it – toasting definitely enhances the flavor.

Ingredients

- 4 Medjool dates soaked in water– reserve water
- 1-cup old-fashioned oats toasted
- 1-teaspoon vegan plant butter coconut butter melted
- 1- teaspoon cinnamon
- ½ teaspoon allspice
- ½ cup walnuts coarsely chopped
- ½ cup dried cranberries
- ¼ cup dried tart cherries
- ¼ cup golden flax seeds
- ¼ cup figs dried Calimyrna figs, coarsely chopped
- 2-tablespoons pomegranate molasses or agave
- 1-tablespoon chia seeds
- 1-teaspoon anise seeds
- 1/8-teaspoon unrefined sea salt

Directions

1. Soak dates in water for at least 30 minutes.
2. Meanwhile, preheat oven to 350° F.
3. Toss oats with plant butter, cinnamon and allspice.
4. Spoon onto parchment lined baking sheet.
5. Bake on center rack of 350° F preheated oven for 10 minutes – stir a couple of times to keep from burning.
6. Remove from oven and cool.
7. Remove dates from water, remove seeds (reserve soaking water).
8. In medium bowl, mash the dates with a fork
9. Add the oats, walnuts, cherries, cranberries, flax seeds, figs, pomegranate molasses, chia seed, anise seeds, cinnamon, allspice and sea salt.
10. Stir and or knead mixture to combine and to form a cohesive dough.
11. If too stiff stir in small amounts of soaking water used for the dates until the mixture holds together.
12. Once the mixture becomes cohesive, let it rest 15 minutes for the chia and flax to absorb some of the moisture and for the flavors to blend.
13. Using a 1 tablespoon cookie scoop pick up mixture then using hands roll into balls.
14. Store in refrigerator for 1 week or freeze up to 1 month.
15. Energy nibbles can also be pressed into an 8" pan lined with parchment then cut into squares.

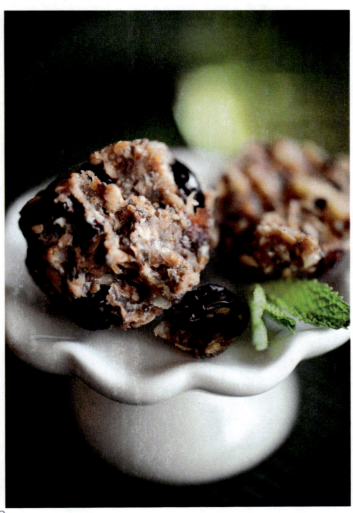

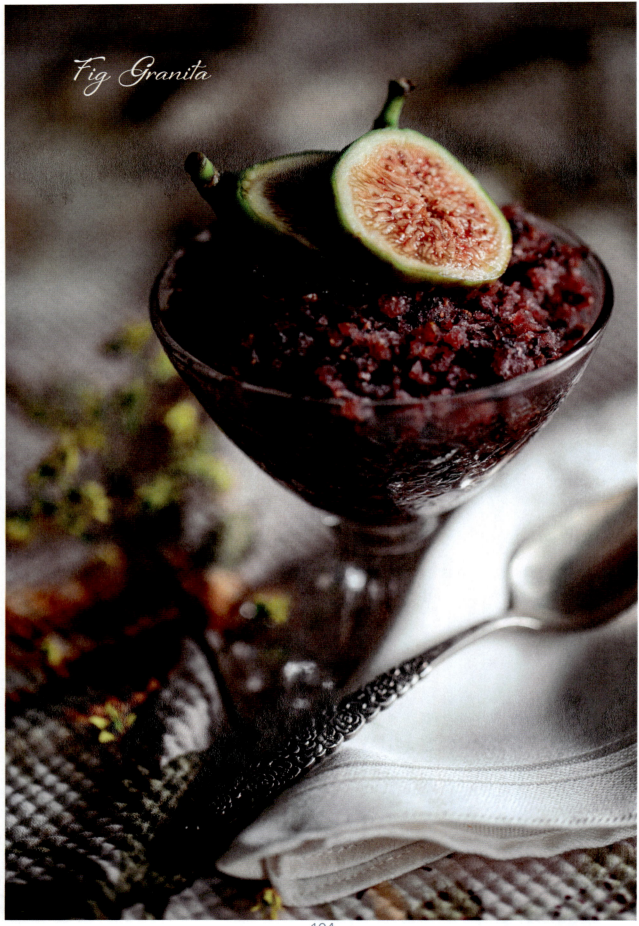

Fig Granita

Makes 4 servings.

Even though granita is an Italian dessert, it's so yummy that I Greek-anized mine with classic ingredients from the Aegean islands - fresh figs, cinnamon & lemon - to make it a stunning mezze. Nóstimo (delicious)!

Ingredients

- 1-pint fresh ripe figs, hard stems removed
- ½ teaspoon lemon zest from organic lemon
- 1-teaspoon fresh lemon juice
- ½ teaspoon ground cinnamon

Directions

1. Wash figs thoroughly with cold water and remove any course stems.
2. Transfer to a blender with lemon zest, lemon juice, and cinnamon.
3. Pulse several times to puree.
4. Pour into a baking dish about ½ inch deep and place in freezer uncovered
5. Freeze until puree just begins to freeze, about 45 minutes.
6. Puree will begin to freeze from the edges but center will still be slushy
7. Using a fork, stir the crystals from the edge of the granita into the center
8. Chill in freezer until granita is almost frozen –
9. Stir, scrape and break up clumps with fork about every 30 minutes for 2 hours or until it becomes light and fluffy.
10. Serve immediately - garnish with fresh figs or store in freezer in covered container.
11. Best if eaten within a week – fluff with fork just before serving.

Nóstimo

"Delicious!"

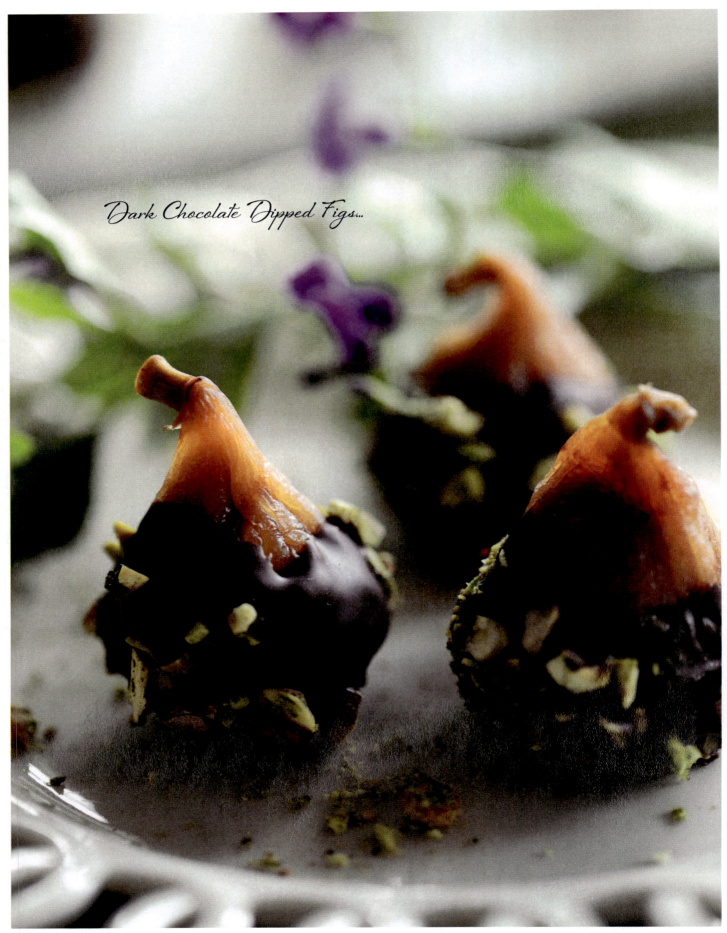

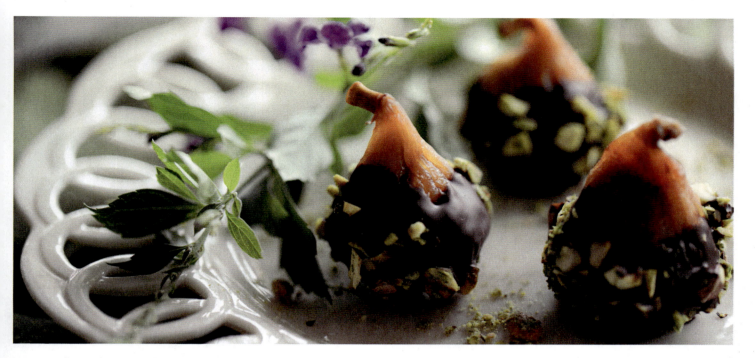

Dark Chocolate Dipped Figs with Pistachios & Anise Dust

Makes 12 to 16 figs.

The tiny amount of ground anise makes these chocolate dipped figs ethereal.

Ingredients

- 3 ounces nondairy dark chocolate bar, chopped
- 12 dried figs
- 2 tablespoons finely chopped pistachios
- ¼ teaspoon ground anise seeds

Directions

1. Press and shape figs with your fingers to plump them up and to form them into a nice shape.
2. Hand chop pistachios together with ground anise seeds – set aside.
3. Chop chocolate into small pieces and place in a small bowl.
4. Fill small pot with 2 to 3 inches of water and bring to a simmer over medium heat.
5. Turn off the burner and place bowl with chocolate over the pot with water to melt.
6. Stir until the chocolate is melted and smooth.
7. Remove bowl from the pan with water and let cool for a couple of minutes.
8. Line a baking sheet with parchment paper.
9. Holding a fig by the stem, dip into the chocolate to coat – let excess chocolate drip back into the bowl.
10. Lightly press the bottom half of fig into chopped pistachios and ground anise – set on parchment paper.
11. Repeat with remaining figs.
12. Let the figs set for 15 minutes in fridge before serving.
13. Will keep 4 to 5 days in the fridge.

Fig Fruit & Nut Salami

Makes 2 salami.

This easy to prepare, plant-based Italian specialty makes a dense, delicious, and interesting mezze. I make mine with Dry Sack Sherry. My mother used inexpensive sherry to marinate nuts and fruits – and they were phenomenal. But I fell in love with Dry Sack at a gourmet cooking class 20 years ago. I like to keep a bottle on hand. It adds a complexity of flavors – a touch of sweet, and a taste of toffee to my fig salami. Williams & Humbert Dry Sack Sherry is plant-based and vegan friendly.

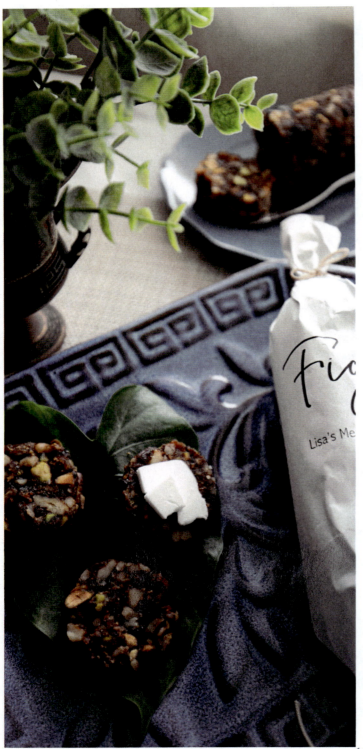

Ingredients

- 10 ounce package Calimyrna dried figs
- 6 pitted medjool dates, seeded
- ½ cup raisins
- 1 cup walnuts
- ½ cup unsalted pistachios
- 2 tablespoons dry sherry or black tea
- 1 teaspoon anise seeds
- ½ teaspoon ground cinnamon
- Optional confectioners' sugar

Directions

1. Remove hard stems from figs and cut in half.
2. Place figs, dates, raisins, walnuts, pistachios, sherry, anise seeds, and cinnamon in food processor fitted with steel blade.
3. Pulse until ingredients are coarsely chopped but still have distinct texture.
4. Divide mixture in half to make 2 salamis.
5. Transfer fig and nut mixture onto hard surface on top of a piece of plastic wrap.
6. The ingredients will be a little sticky – wrap each half with plastic wrap – roll into smooth salami shape.
7. The salami can be served immediately, but tastes best if it's allowed to cure for a day or two.
8. Just before serving, roll in optional confectioners' sugar. Slice into thin rounds with a serated knife and serve with plant-based feta or other plant-based cheese.
9. It's best to cut the salami when it's cold with a sharp serrated knife.
10. Store in refrigerator, covered with plastic wrap in Ziploc bag.
11. The Italians say fig salami will last throughout the winter holiday season.

Fruit with Almond Cream Syrup & Yogurt

This beautiful and delicious mezze is perfect for midmorning brunch, or as a light dessert to enjoy anytime. I serve it topped with fruit and nuts. But it also makes a mouthwatering fruit dip for a fruit platter.

Ingredients

- Fruit of choice
- A few almonds, pistachios, or walnuts
- Equal amounts of "Almond Cream Syrup" on page 134 and plain or vanilla nondairy yogurt such as Kite Hill brand

Directions

1. Wash and prep the fruit – I used fresh figs and frozen wild blueberries thawed.
2. Coarsely chop nuts.
3. In a small bowl, whisk together equal amounts of the Almond Cream Syrup and nondairy yogurt.
4. Spoon the Almond Cream Syrup and yogurt onto bottom of serving bowl or plate.
5. Arrange fruit on top and sprinkle with nuts.

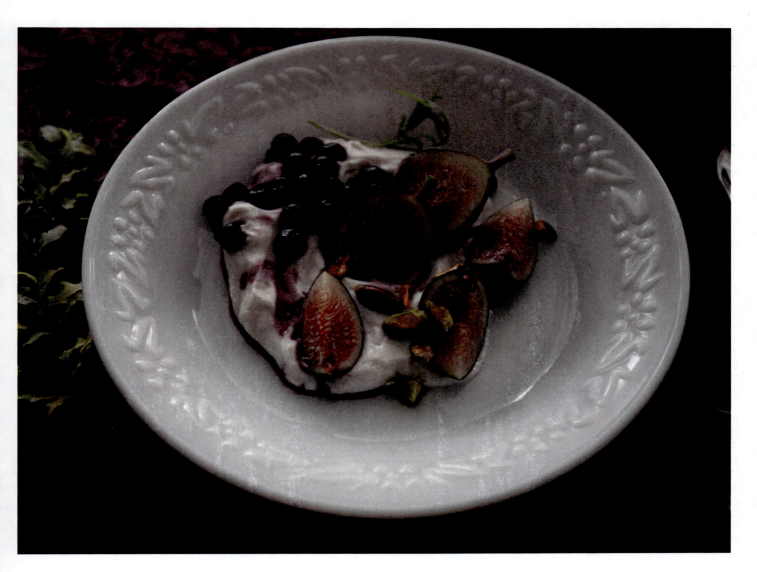

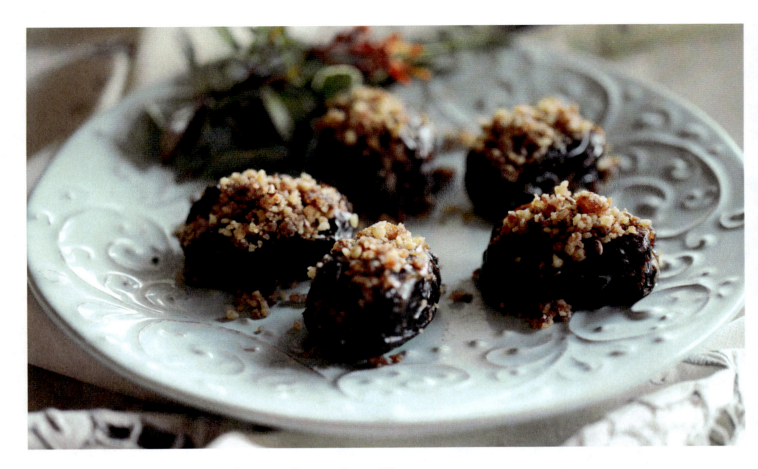

Medjool Dates with Walnut Stuffing

Makes 8 mezze portions.

My yia yia had a date tree in her yard that was outside of her kitchen window. Her fresh dates never made it to a mezze platter because we ate them fresh, plucked from the heavy clusters that hung from the tree. To me - they were, and still are a heavenly, sweet delicacy. Sometimes I crave something sweet, and a humble date provides that perfect taste of happiness. Plus, it nourishes my body with fiber, iron, and potassium.

A few years back when I took a raw-food cooking course, I was introduced to Medjool dates. Medjools aka Joolies - elevate the fruit to a new level. Medjools are larger than other dates in the market. When fresh, their plump pulp is moist and creamy. They make a whole-food plant-based mezze that's near nirvana.

Ingredients

- 9 whole Medjool dates
- 1½ cup walnuts
- ½ teaspoon whole golden flax seeds
- ¼ teaspoon ground cinnamon
- Pinch of unrefined sea salt

Directions

1. Slice down the center of the dates lengthwise.
2. Remove the seeds.
3. Place 1 date in food processor with walnuts, flax seeds, cinnamon, and salt.
4. Pulse until finely ground.
5. Spoon and lightly pressed ground nuts into the cut.
6. Ready to serve but will keep for a week covered in the fridge.

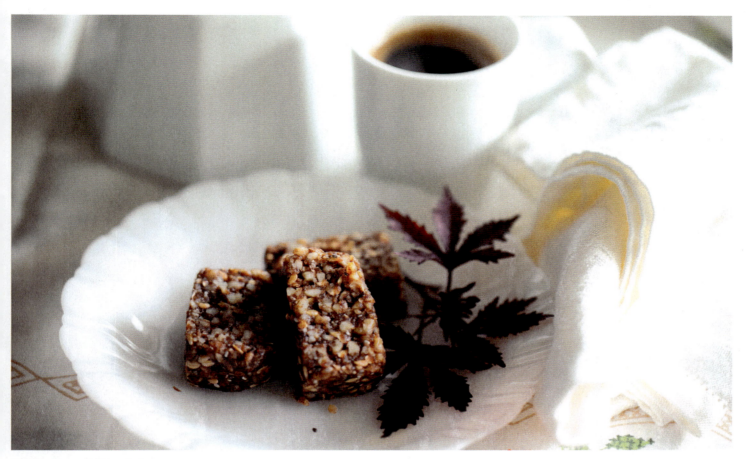

Naked Baklava

Makes 8 mezze portions.

Ingredients

- 1 cup walnuts
- 2 medjool dates, seeded
- 1 teaspoon ground cinnamon
- ¼ teaspoon ground cloves
- 1 teaspoon agave nectar
- 1 teaspoon chia seeds
- 1 tablespoon golden flax seeds
- Pinch of unrefined sea salt

Directions

1. In food processor, add the walnuts, dates, cinnamon, cloves, agave, and salt.
2. Pulse until walnuts are coarsely chopped and mixture is blended.
3. Transfer mixture to small bowl – knead in chia and flax seeds with hands.
4. Place mixture onto chopping board and form into a 6-inch log, flatten top to form a rectangle.
5. Slice rectangle in half and slice halves into 4 pieces.
6. Store in refrigerator up to 1 week.

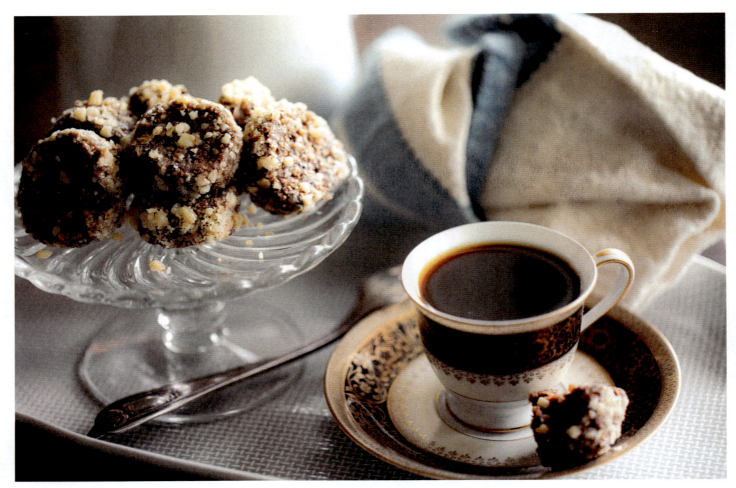

Naked Fig & Nut Cookie Bites - Skaltsounia

Makes 12 to 16 mezze cookies.

Traditional skaltsounia are Christmas cookies stuffed with a dried fruit and nut filling. This is my modern, naked take on that Greek pastry. It's a guilt and gluten free way to enjoy a rich and complex flavored, not too sweet confection without the fuss of making cookie dough. It makes a delicious sweetmeat on a holiday mezze table. Note: if figs and/or dates are very dry, soak whole fruit in warm coffee or water for 15 minutes. Drain well and proceed with recipe..

Ingredients

- 8 dried Calimyrna figs coarsely chopped
- 2 medjool dates pitted
- ½ apple with peel coarsely chopped
- ¼ cup golden or dark raisins
- 1 cup walnuts
- 2 ounces dark chocolate grated
- 1 teaspoon instant coffee or espresso powder
- 2 tablespoons chia seeds
- ½ teaspoon cinnamon
- 1/8 teaspoon ground cloves
- Zest from 1 organic orange

Directions

1. Place all ingredients into food processor.
2. Pulse until chopped and blended but not pureed.
3. Transfer mixture to a bowl and cover with plastic wrap.
4. Chill the mixture for an 1 hour or longer.
5. Roll the dough into 2 logs about 8-inches long each.
6. Cut each log into 8 round pieces.
7. Dust with additional walnut crumbs, cinnamon and/or confectioner's sugar.
8. Store in a Ziploc or covered container in the refrigerator for up to a week.

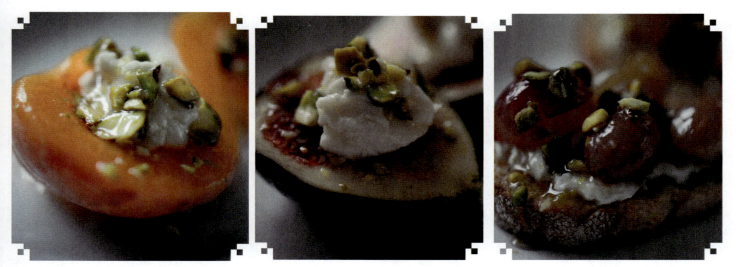

Roasted Apricot　　　Roasted Fresh Fig　　　Roasted Grapes

Roasted Fruit with Balsamic Cinnamon Syrup

Makes approximately 1 dozen apricots or figs or a pint of other fruit.

My daughter and son-in-law love to try out local trendy cafes and bistros. She tells me frequently that no fruit dessert compares with the delicious flavor of my roasted fruits with Balsamic Cinnamon Syrup.

Ingredients
- Fruit of your choice like fresh apricots, fresh figs, strawberries, grapes, etc.
- ¼ cup "Balsamic Cinnamon Syrup" on page 143
- 2 tablespoons agave nectar

Directions
1. Prepare the Balsamic Cinnamon Syrup ahead and cool to room temperature.
2. Preheat oven to 375°F.
3. Cut fruit(s) into halves.
4. In medium bowl toss the fruit with Balsamic Syrup and agave.
5. Line a baking sheet with parchment paper.
6. Pour the fruit halves with syrup onto the baking sheet – arrange fruit in one layer.
7. Place the baking sheet with fruit on center rack of preheated oven.
8. Roast for approximately 15 minutes or until the fruit softens.
9. Remove from oven and cool to room temperature.
10. The fruits are scrumptious on their own. But you may want to try topping them with plant-based cream cheese or feta, sprinkle with chopped pistachios, and drizzle with accumulated syrup and/or additional Balsamic Cinnamon Syrup.
11. Serve at room temperature or chilled.
12. Store covered in the refrigerator for 3 or 4 days.

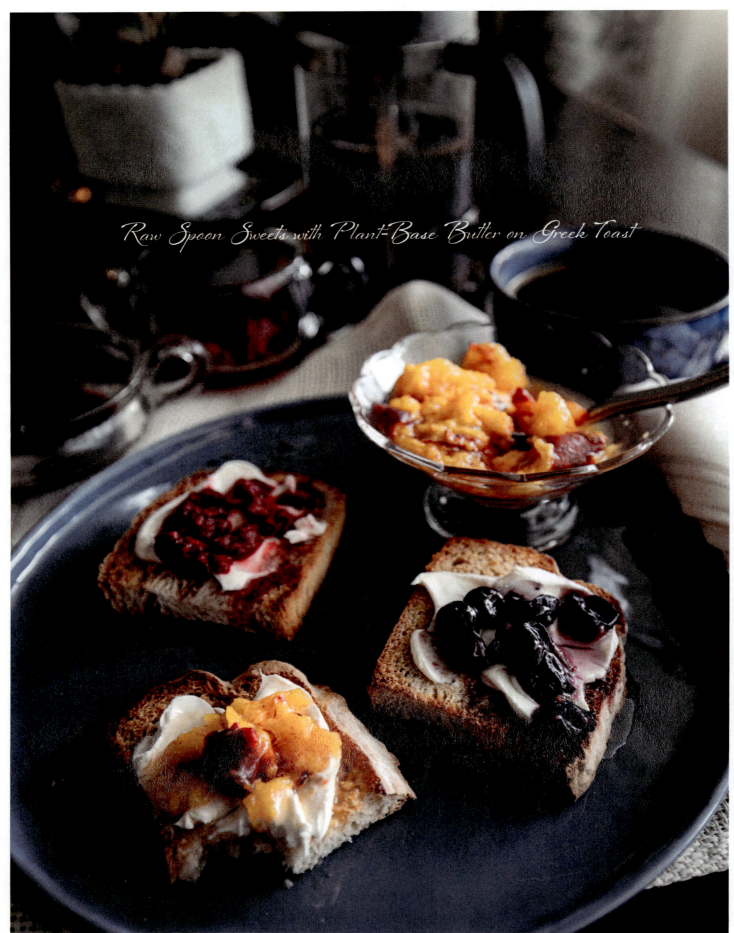

Raw Spoon Sweets with Plant-Base Butter on Greek Toast

Spoon Sweets for a New Day

Raw spoon sweets make a beautiful breakfast mezze table. In addition to toast, serve the spoon sweets with nondairy yogurt (Kite Hill brand is excellent). They're also fantastic as a topping for steel-cut oats, on top of pancakes, or simply stirred into a glass of cold spring water.

Spoon sweets are just what their name states — spoons of sweet. They are usually some sort of fruit cooked in heavy, sugary syrup. But in addition to fruits, other whole foods such as nuts, rose petals, eggplants, and even mastic tree gum were transformed into spoon sweets. My mother told us yia yia, in her younger years, made delicate orange blossom and geranium leaf spoon sweets from plants in her yard.

Making preserves takes skill and patience. The cook's challenge is to maintain the food's original wholeness and firm texture. This is accomplished by a slow, gentle cooking process passed down from mother to daughter through the generations. The preparation of spoon sweets could take many hours or even a couple of days. Traditionally it was served on cake or just on a spoon to visitors as a gesture of hospitality. My father loved it best, stirred into a glass of cold water.

When I was a child, most spoon sweets were homemade but not at our house — because my mother was ahead of her time and was concerned about the substantial sugar content. So we depended on the occasional gift of the precious preserves from family and friends. Even then, she would only allow a rare taste of the sweet as a dessert. My father, on the other hand, had a deep affection for the candied confection. Somehow, from somewhere, he could magically produce a jar of his beloved Grecian delicacy. Hidden from the site of our mother — he would sneak us syrupy spoonfuls of sinfulness.

To be honest, I always found the preserves to be so sweet that the fruit's flavor was muted. But no preserves can come close to the beauty of a glass jar jammed packed with a perfectly prepared fruit.

I know sugar can cause health problems. Like my father, I also know that life is too short not to share an occasional taste of sweet. But my mother's wisdom inspired me to come up with a healthier, simpler, and what I believe to be an even tastier version of spoon sweet.

One of my first cooking certificates was from Matthew Kenney's Culinary Academy. Raw foods are full of enzymes, making the food's health benefits more bio-available — more accessible for the body to utilize. I love to mash, slice, shred, or chop fresh raw fruits like berries, apples, bananas - almost any fruit, to serve on toasted Greek bread, flatbread, or pita. If the fruit is not sweet enough for your taste, drizzle it with a little raw agave. Brighten it up with a few drops of lemon and sprinkle with a bit of cinnamon or allspice. Nuts also make a healthy, tasty spoon sweet.

Ingredients

- Raw or frozen fruit(s) and nut(s) of your choice
- Agave
- Pinch of cinnamon

Directions

1. Coarsely mash fruit with a fork.
2. Drizzle on a little agave nectar and sprinkle with a little cinnamon.
3. Or - try drizzling with a little Balsamic Cinnamon Syrup.
4. Serve on toast, pancakes, oatmeal, or stirred into an icy cold glass of water.

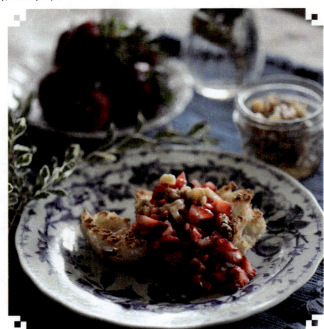

Strawberry Spoon Sweet
& Wet Walnuts on Greek Toast

Roasted Pumpkin Spoon Sweet

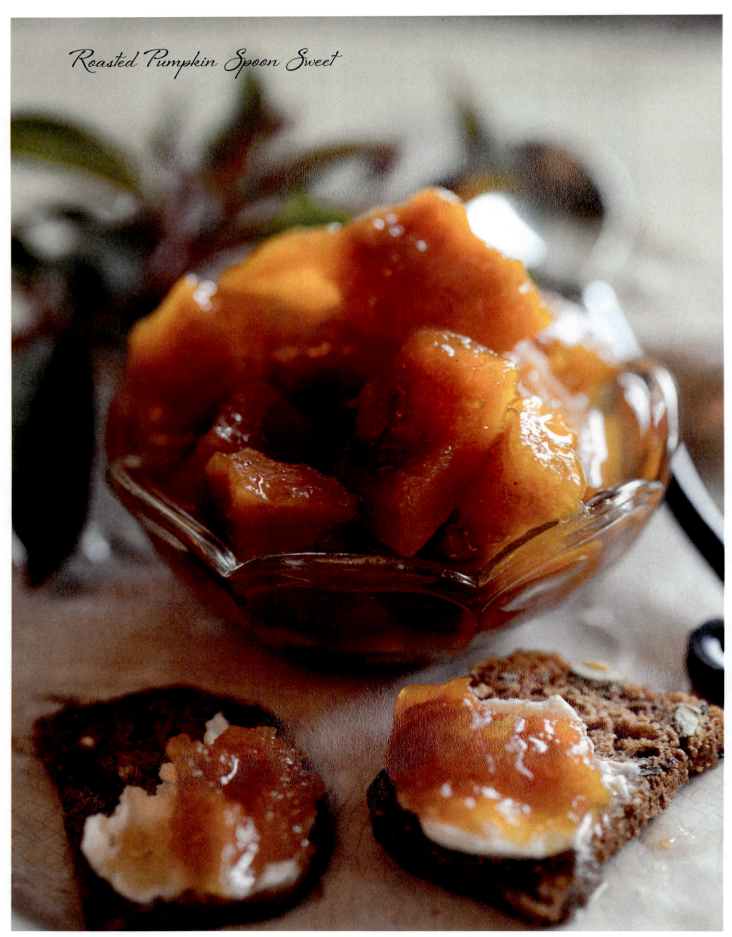

Roasted Pumpkin Spoon Sweet Recipe

Yields approximately 1 pint jar full of spoon sweet with syrup.

This makes an extra special mezze to offer as a gesture of sweet hospitality, especially during the holiday season. It embodies the delicious flavors of fall and winter.

Spoon sweets are traditionally simmered in syrup on top of the stove. But roasting enriches the pumpkin flavor and its toothsome texture. This pumpkin spoon sweet adds a punch of autumn color for a mezze brunch, or luscious spoon of sweet for a visitor. It's exceptional on toast, yogurt, stirred into barley or oatmeal. It also makes a tasty and unique confection to serve with breakfast on a Thanksgiving or Christmas morning.

Several winter squashes are interchangeable with pumpkins. Even famous brands of canned "pumpkin" are not actually made from pumpkins, but something closer to a butternut or Hubbard squash. The flesh of these winter squashes are richer in color, sweetness, and texture. So I use butternut squash to make my oven-roasted "pumpkin" spoon sweet.

Ingredients

- 1 small butternut squash around 2- 2 ½ pounds
- ¾ cup raw sugar
- ¼ teaspoon ground pumpkin pie spice
- 2 tablespoons plant-based whiskey – like Ballentine's Scotch Whiskey
- 1 tablespoon spring or filtered water
- ½ teaspoon fresh lemon juice

Directions

1. Wash the squash and peel – make sure to remove all of the hard peel.
2. Cut the squash in half and scoop out the seeds with a spoon.
3. Cut the halves into 1-inch pieces and place in a large glass casserole dish.
4. Using a coffee grinder, pulse the sugar with pumpkin pie spice to break down the sugar crystals.
5. Sprinkle the squash cubes with sugar mixture, stir in the whiskey, and water – stir to coat the squash pieces and set aside loosely covered with foil for 1 hour. The sugar will dissolve and squash will weep.
6. Preheat the oven to 300° F.
7. Using a spoon, toss the squash pieces once again before transferring to the oven.
8. Keep the loose foil over the casserole dish.
9. Bake pumpkin on center rack of 300° F preheated oven - for 1 hour stirring half way through.
10. After 1 hour, stir the squash to coat with the pan syrup, and turn the oven off.
11. Stir in the lemon juice and let the squash cool to room temperature in the oven to reabsorb some of the syrup.
12. Store in a covered glass jar in the fridge for up to 3 days.

Loukoumades with Flax Seeds & Greek Coffee Glaze

Makes about 2-dozen

Ingredients

- 1-1/2 cups unbleached bread flour
- ½ cup whole-wheat pastry flour
- 2 tablespoons golden flax seeds ground in coffee grinder to a fine powder
- 2 teaspoons instant yeast
- ¼ teaspoon sea salt
- 1 cup lukewarm filtered or bottled water
- 1-teaspoon vanilla
- Extra light olive oil for frying

Directions Loukoumades

1. In large bowl, whisk together bread flour, whole-wheat pastry flour, ground flax seed, yeast and salt.
2. Stir water and vanilla into flour mixture to make soft, sticky dough.
3. Cover bowl with plastic wrap and set aside in warm place to rise for 1 hour or until doubled.
4. Heat oil in skillet over medium heat.
5. Spray a spoon with non-stick spray.
6. Scoop up dough with coated spoon and drop into hot oil.
7. Cook and turn puffs with slotted spoon until golden on all sides.
8. Drain on paper towels.
9. Dip loukoumades into coffee icing.
10. Serve immediately.
11. Alternatively: sprinkle with confectioners sugar or split open and spread with spoon sweets or preserves.

Greek Coffee Glaze

Ingredients

- 1 cup powdered sugar
- 2 tablespoons Greek coffee or strong American coffee
- 1/8-teaspoon ground cinnamon

Directions

1. In small bowl, whisk all ingredients together.
2. Drizzle on Loukoumades.

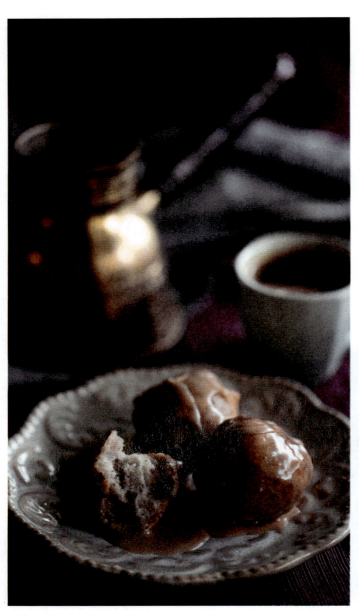

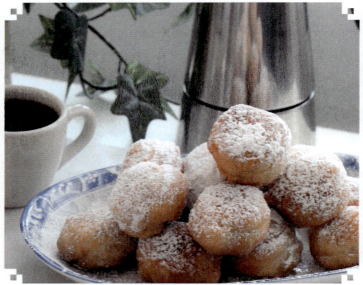

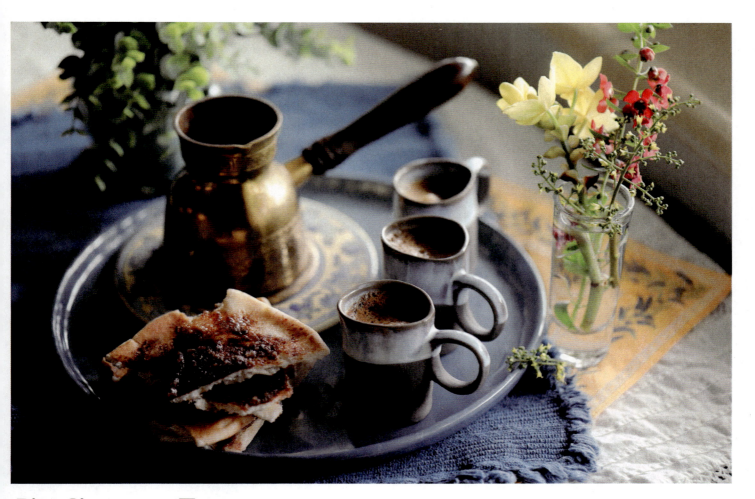

Pita Cinnamon Toast

Each pita provides 4 to 8 mezze servings

These are simple, a little sinful, and fantastically delicious! Serve them with Greek or American coffee, fruit, nondairy yogurt, and nuts - for a quick mezze brunch.

Ingredients

- 1 - 8-inch pita or flat bread
- 2 teaspoons plant based butter softened

Directions

1. Preheat broiler..
2. Spread plant based butter all over the concave or under side of the pita and place buttered side up on baking sheet.
3. Place baking sheet on center rack of oven with door ajar so you can have a peek in.
4. Broil pita on center rack for 1 to 3 minutes – I watch mine closely to see the edges turn golden and butter become bubbly.
5. Remove from oven and immediately sprinkle with 2 teaspoons cinnamon sugar while pita is hot and butter is bubbly.
6. Serve immediately or at room temperature – I hand tear mine into quarters or eighths – if you prefer uniform pieces, place the pita on a cutting board - use a pizza wheel or knife to cut into strips or wedges.

Cinnamon Sugar

- Whisk 1/4 cup raw cane sugar with 2 teaspoons cinnamon.
- Store any leftovers in small Ziploc.

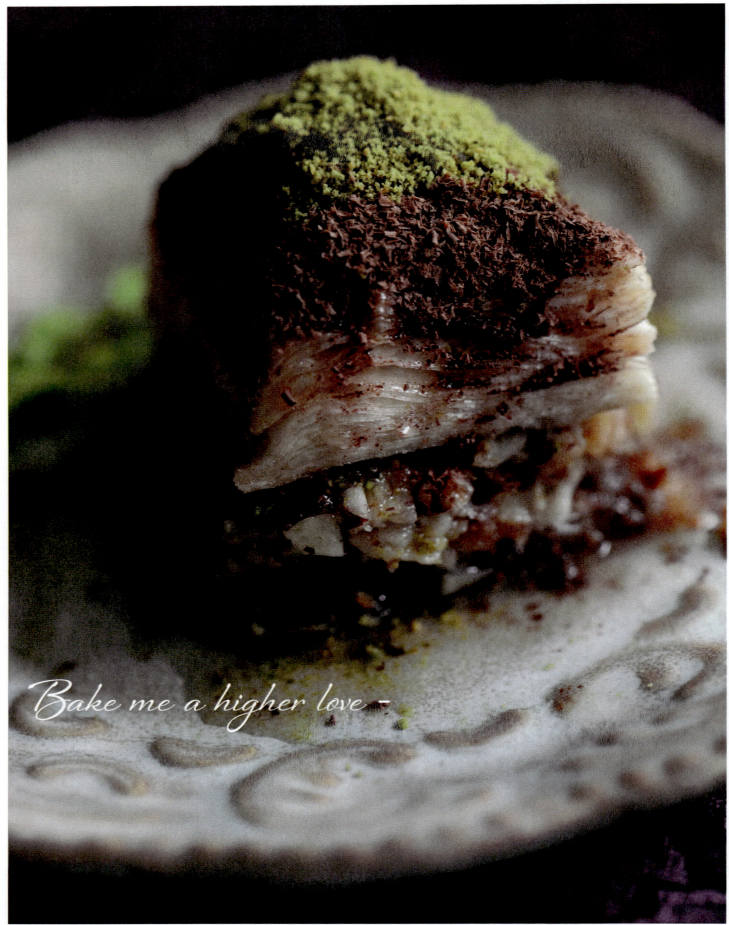

Bake me a higher love -

Baklava with Spiced Almond Milk Syrup & Bitter Dark Chocolate

Makes 24 to 32 squares.

This is my take on Turkish Sutlu Bitter Baklava. It's a unique baklava recipe with sublime flavor and elegant allure. It's plant based, sweetened with cinnamon almond milk syrup, topped with dark chocolate shavings, and finished with ground pistachios. It's an "amen" on a plate.

This recipe makes a large pan of baklava. Enough for a large mezze gathering and leftovers to share with friends and neighbors.

Ingredients

- 16 ounce package frozen phyllo dough
- ½ cup plant-based butter
- ½ cup olive oil
- ½ pound walnuts coarsely chopped
- ½ pound almonds coarsely chopped
- 3.7 oz. bar, nondairy dark chocolate
- ½ cup pistachios very finely chopped

Directions for baklava

1. Preheat oven to 325° F.
2. Pulse nuts in food processor until fine crumbs form – do not over process into a nut butter.
3. Melt butter in small saucepan over low heat.
4. Remove melted butter from stove – add olive oil and stir to blend.
5. With pastry brush paint the bottom of a 9x13 pan with olive oil and butter mixture.
6. Lay a phyllo sheet on bottom of pan - brush with melted mixture.
7. Repeat with approximately half of the of phyllo sheets, lightly buttering every 2nd to 3rd sheet.
8. Evenly sprinkle the nut mixture onto the top of the buttered layers.
9. Top nut mixture with remaining phyllo sheets very lightly brushing every 2nd to 3rd sheet with melted butter mixture.
10. With very sharp knife cut baklava into small squares making sure to cut through to the bottom of the pan.
11. Pour any remaining butter and olive oil mixture into the cuts.
12. Bake on the center rack of preheated oven for 1 hour – or until golden brown.
13. Remove from oven, spoon 1 cup of cooled Almond Milk Syrup onto hot pastry making sure to spoon into cuts.
14. Cool the baklava to room temperature before topping with chocolate and pistachios.
15. Using a microplane grate dark chocolate onto the top of the baklava.
16. Sprinkle with finely chopped pistachios and offer remaining syrup for guests to drizzle over their baklava.

Spiced Almond Milk Syrup

Ingredients

- 1 cup plain, unsweetened almond milk homemade or store bought
- 1 cup raw cane sugar
- ¼ cup spring or filtered water
- 1 cinnamon stick
- ½ teaspoon pure vanilla extract

Directions Almond Milk Syrup

1. Add almond milk, sugar, water, and cinnamon stick to small saucepan.
2. Bring to a rolling boil over medium heat and boil for 3 minutes.
3. Reduce heat to low and simmer the syrup uncovered for 15 minutes.
4. Remove from stove and stir in vanilla.
5. Cool to room temperature and remove cinnamon stick before pouring onto baklava.
6. Store sealed with plastic wrap at room temperature for up to 2 days.

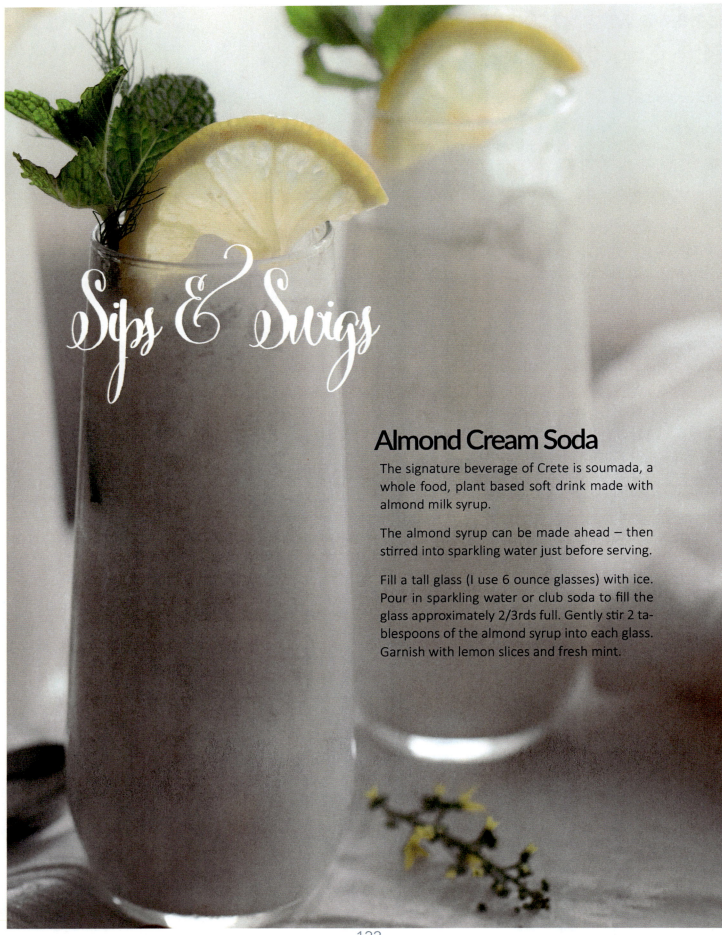

Sips & Swigs

Almond Cream Soda

The signature beverage of Crete is soumada, a whole food, plant based soft drink made with almond milk syrup.

The almond syrup can be made ahead – then stirred into sparkling water just before serving.

Fill a tall glass (I use 6 ounce glasses) with ice. Pour in sparkling water or club soda to fill the glass approximately 2/3rds full. Gently stir 2 tablespoons of the almond syrup into each glass. Garnish with lemon slices and fresh mint.

Greek Coffee

A research article in SAGE Journal indicates a connection between chronic boiled Greek coffee consumption and longevity. Greek coffee is ground to a fine powder. When it is boiled on low heat, the coffee releases polyphenols and antioxidants. The Greek island, Ikaria, takes pride in the fact that its elders live longer than any other place in the world – and scientists believe the secret to their longevity may be due to daily ingestion of Greek coffee.

Greek coffee is very different from American coffee. Greek coffee is brought just to the boil then served in a small cup WITH the grounds.

For guests who may be tasting Greek coffee for the first time, they may want to try a cup with sugar. Also, it's tradition to allow the coffee to sit for a couple of minutes to allow the grounds to settle to the bottom of the cup. The coffee is then consumed with small sips.

Ingredients

- 1 heaping teaspoon of ground Greek coffee for each espresso or demitasse cup
- A demitasse cup full of spring or filtered water for each cup
- Depending on how many coffees you're making, you will need the appropriate size Greek coffee pot – known as briki. Brikia usually come in 1, 2, 4, and 6 cup sizes. They're sold on Amazon.
- Raw cane sugar to your taste: no sugar (sketos), ½ teaspoon sugar (me oligi), 1 teaspoon sugar (metrios), 2 teaspoons sugar (glykis)
- Note: I like to blitz the sugar in a coffee grinder, blender, or food processor until it's powdery before stirring it into my coffee. It makes a frothier coffee.

Directions

1. Fill the espresso or demitasse cup(s) with water.
2. Pour the water into the briki (Greek coffee pot).
3. Stir to blend and dissolve the sugar – and don't stir again.
4. Place the briki on a medium low heat.
5. Bring the coffee to a boil – do not leave the pot – you need to be attentive so the coffee doesn't boil over.
6. As the coffee begins to boil, froth will start to rise from the center of the briki, remove from briki from the stove.
7. If making more than 1 cup, spoon equal amounts of the froth into each cup then slowly pour the remaining coffee into cups.

It's traditional to serve Greek coffee with a glass of cold water.

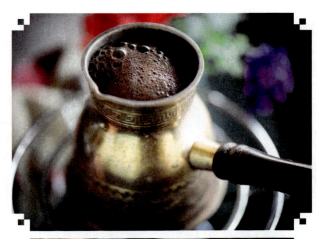

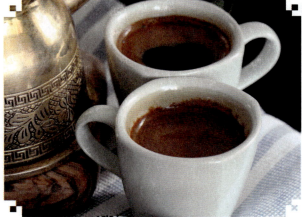

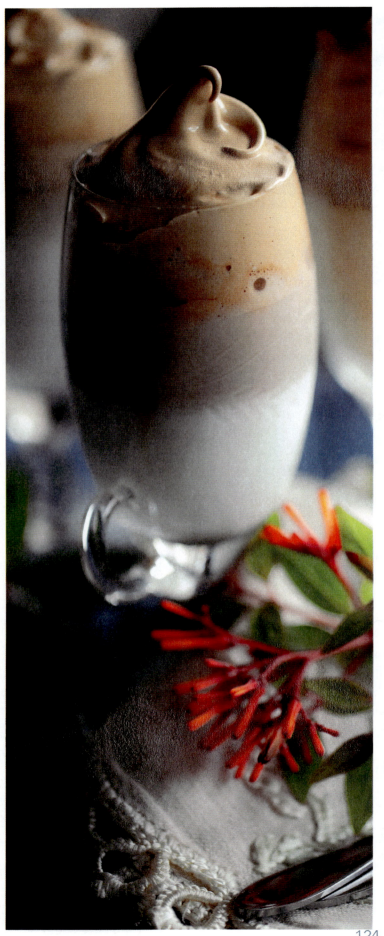

Greek Whipped Coffee Frappe

Makes 4 to 6 servings.

The most popular coffee drink served in Greece is a frappé. They are made with Nescafé, an instant coffee powder. Frappés are served cold with optional milk and sugar.

The Koreans came up with Dalonga whipped coffee. It was created during the pandemic to keep people in isolation. It's also know as "quarantine coffee". It looked so delicious that I had to come up with a Greek version by whipping Nescafé instant coffee with raw cane sugar, water, and vanilla using an electric mixer. This makes a light, coffee topping for a cold and creamy treat. Because of the sugar content, I offer it as an after mezze dessert and use small, 4-ounce glasses. If you prefer, you could substitute regular or espresso instant coffee for the Nescafé. If you're up for a luscious treat, this is a must try!

Ingredients

- 3 tablespoons raw cane sugar ground to a powder in a blender or coffee grinder
- 2 tablespoons Nescafe Frappe instant coffee
- 2 tablespoons cool water
- ½ teaspoon pure vanilla extract

Directions

1. Use a coffee grinder (blender or food processor) to blitz the raw cane sugar into a powder.
2. Place the powdered cane sugar in a small bowl together with the Nescafe Frappe instant coffee, water, and vanilla.
3. Using an electric mixer starting on low, mix the ingredients until blended.
4. Increase mixer speed to high and whip the coffee mixture until it turns light, creamy, and holds its shape.
5. Fill small (I used 4-ounce) cups about 2/3rds full with cold nondairy milk, then heap dollops of whipped coffee on top.
6. Serve with small espresso spoons to stir and blend the whipped coffee frappe with the milk.

Horta & Beet Liqueur Shots

Makes 1 to 2 tablespoon shots.

A shot of horta (greens juice) or beet liqueur can upgrade the vitamins, minerals, prebiotics, antioxidants, iron, and conversation at mezze gatherings.

If you don't have a juicer, used juicers are often available at thrift stores. I picked up a top of the line Hurom brand for $50. But I've seen other good brands, including Breville, for much less. I don't use my juicer daily, but it's nice to have it when I'm craving green juice or for special recipes.

I did make daily green juice or green smoothie shots for the friars. I kept their portions to about 2 tablespoons each. I also kept a small palate of wheatgrass in the fridge. One of my holistic instructors taught that chewing on a pinched off knob of wheatgrass offered many health benefits. Wheatgrass has a mild sweet taste. But the grass blades can be very fibrous. After you've chewed out all the green goodness, spit out the spent grass.

Ingredients for Horta Shots

- 4 kale leaves or 8 dandelion leaves with stems
- A small handful of wheat grass
- 4 sprigs Italian parsley
- 2 celery ribs
- 1-inch knob of turmeric
- 1 apple – for sweetness, remove seeds and stem

DIRECTIONS

1. Place kale or dandelion leaves, parsley sprigs, celery, turmeric, and apple through juicer.
2. The juice is healthiest if consumed within 15 minutes.

Beet Liqueur Shot

Beets are very sweet so only serve a tablespoon or less. Serve chilled beet brine from homemade or store bought beets in a shot glass.

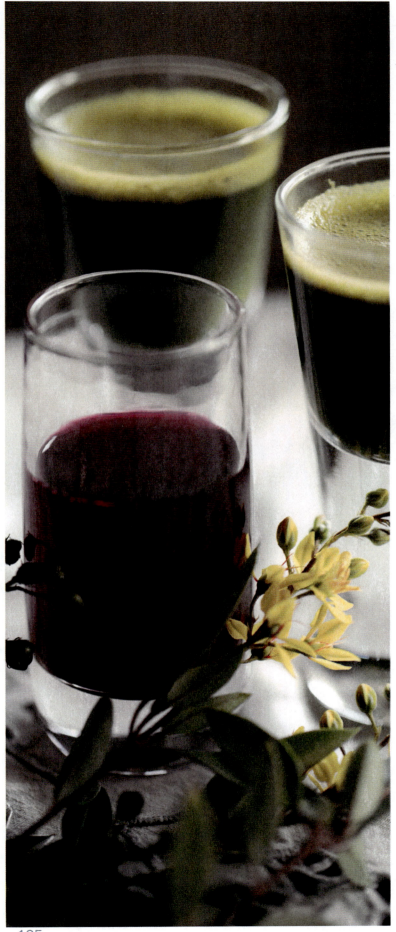

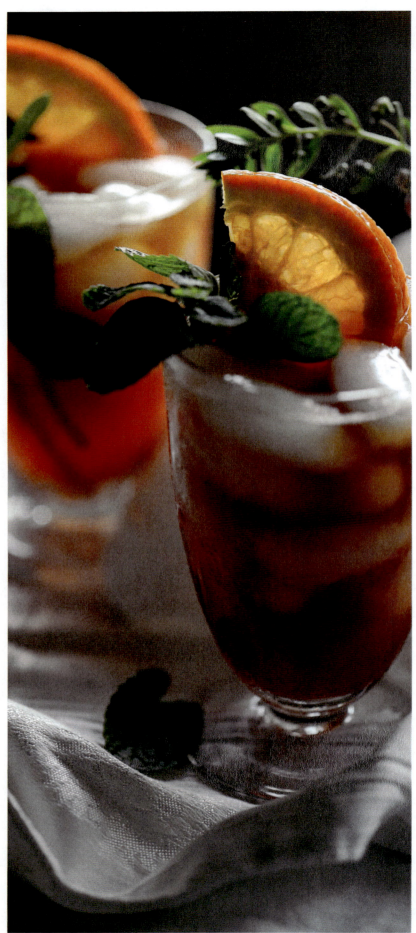

Iced Orange Tea with Cinnamon & Mint

Makes 6 or more servings.

This recipe makes a lightly sweetened and deliciously refreshing iced tea. It's easy to make but takes time for the steeping process to infuse orange, mint, and cinnamon notes. It makes a beautiful and memorable beverage for your mezze table.

Ingredients

- 1 cinnamon stick
- *¼ cup cane sugar (*see note)
- 6 cups boiling spring or filtered water
- 4 of your favorite black tea bags (I used Lipton organic)
- 2 organic oranges sliced into thin rounds, reserve a few slices for garnish
- 3 fresh mint sprigs plus a sprig to garnish each glass
- 1 tablespoon fresh lemon juice

Directions

1. Add a cinnamon stick, sugar, and 6 cups of water to a medium pot – bring to a boil and boil for 5 minutes.
2. Remove the pot from the heat – add 4 tea bags, orange slices, and mint sprigs.
3. Cool the tea until it comes to room temperature.
4. Stir in fresh lemon juice and chill in refrigerator at least 3 hours or overnight.
5. Strain the tea into an ice filled pitcher.
6. Garnish each serving with a fresh orange slice and mint sprig.

*Note: for an extra flavorful mezze beverage, omit the sugar and serve the tea with "Mint & Cinnamon Simple Syrup" on page 143. Serve the syrup on the side and provide each guest a spoon so they can sweeten their tea to their personal taste.

Shepherd's Tea or Mountain Tea

Makes 2 to 4 servings

Made from the stems and flowers of a native plant that thrives on the mountain sides of Greece. Greek mountain tea is rich in antioxidants and polyphenols. Drink it hot or iced, plain or sweetened with agave or honey. My favorite brand is Klio.

Ingredients

- 2 cups of spring or filtered water
- Small handful of tea stems, buds, and flowers
- Agave or honey
- Lemon wedges

Directions

1. Place water and tea in a small saucepan with a lid.
2. Bring to a boil over medium heat and boil with lid ajar for 3 to 5 minutes – the longer it boils, the stronger the tea.
3. Remove from stove and steep covered another 3 to 5 minutes.
4. Strain and serve hot or iced with agave or honey, and lemon wedges.

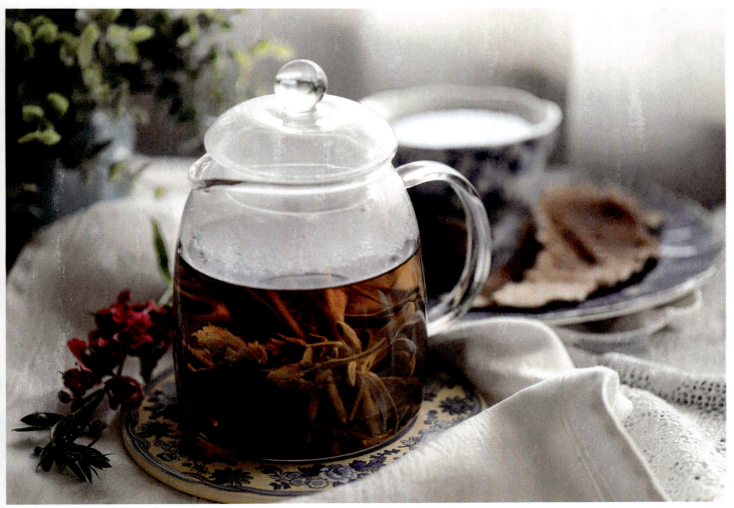

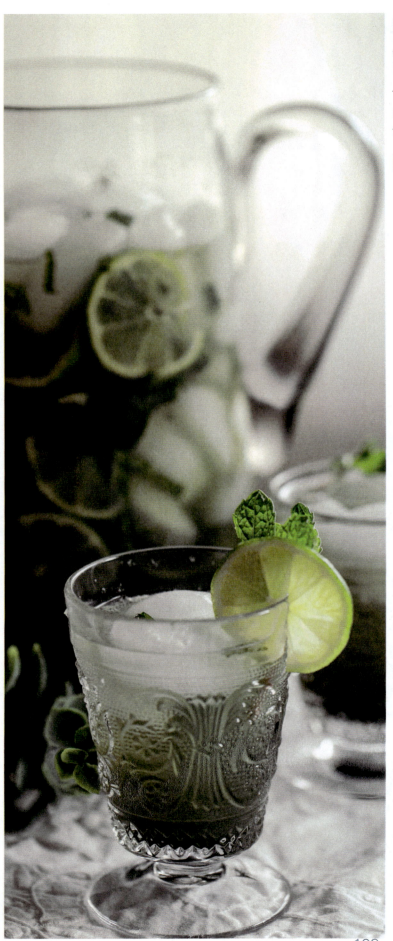

Sparkling Mint Punch with Wheatgrass

This recipe makes a small, 2 quart pitcher of punch. Enough for 6 to 10 mezze sippers. Pretty and perfect for small gatherings.

Ingredients

- 2 quart pitcher (1/2 gallon pitcher)
- 1/4 cup fresh lime juice
- 1 recipe "Mint & Cinnamon Simple Syrup" on page 143
- Ice cubes
- 32 ounces chilled fizzy water like seltzer or soda stream
- Optional: 2 tablespoons fresh juiced wheatgrass, juiced greens, or 1 tablespoon greens powder
- 1 lime cut into thin slices for garnish
- 1 small bunch of mint coarsely chopped for garnish

Directions

1. Mix lime juice and Mint Syrup together in pitcher.
2. Fill pitcher with ice cubes.
3. Pour in seltzer water, and add lime slices, mint, and optional wheatgrass, greens juice, or greens powder
4. Stir to blend - serve immediately.

Green Sips

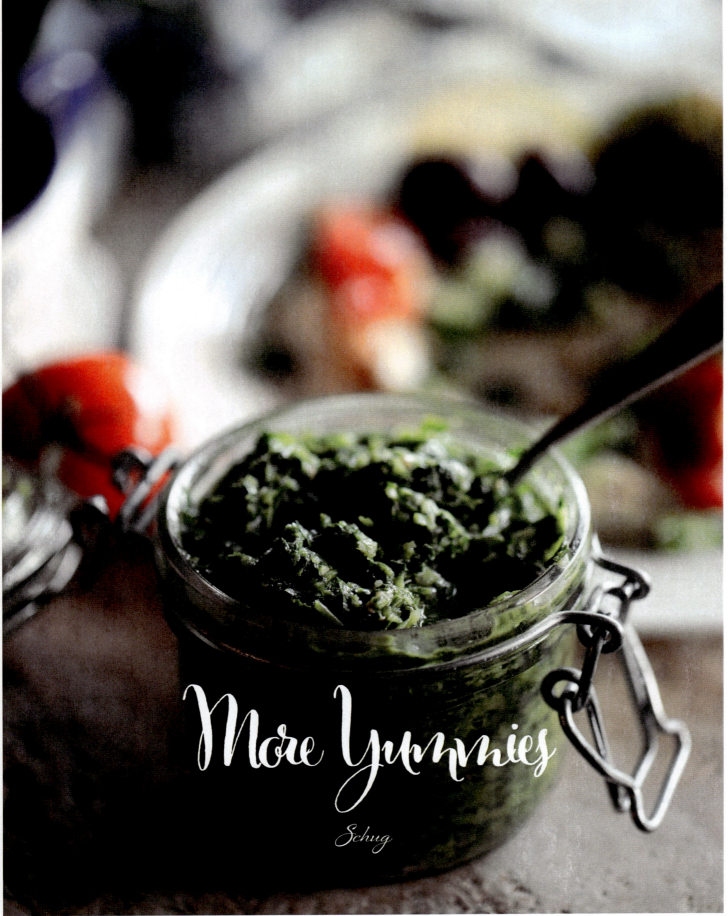

More Yummies

Schug

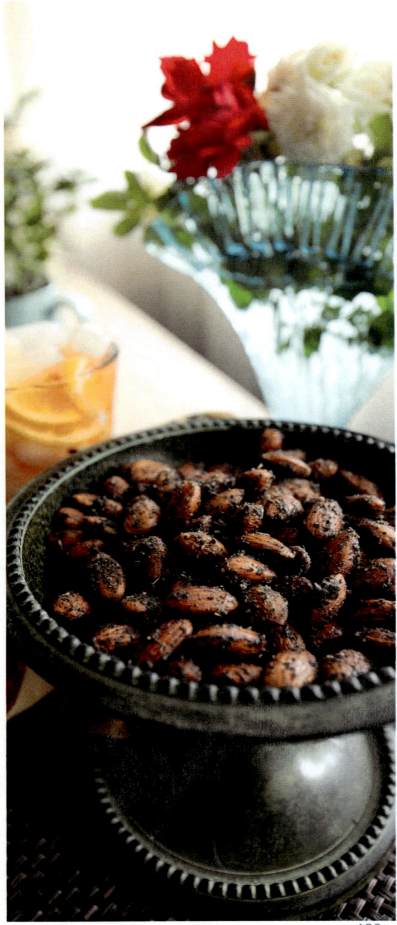

Air Fried Almonds with Greek Seasoning

Makes 1 cup of almonds.

Almonds are common in Greek cooking. They are also symbolic of good luck – that's why candy coated almonds are given to guests at Greek weddings. In my holistic nursing studies I learned just how healthy almonds are – I also learned that much of the nutritional benefit is located in the almond's skin. Once the skin is removed, the almond is no longer considered a whole food. And so, I always buy almonds with the skin intact. This knowledge may also inspire you to make your own almond milk.

Ingredients

- 1 cups raw almonds with skin
- 1-tablespoon olive oil
- 1-tablespoon "Greek Seasoning Blend" on page 142

Directions for Air Frying

1. In a small bowl, mix almonds with olive oil and Greek Seasoning Blend
2. Transfer almonds to basket in air fryer and air fry at 300° for 8 minutes.
3. Remove from fryer and cool completely.
4. Serve at room temperature.
5. Will keep in Ziploc bag for up to 3 days.

Oven Roasted Almonds with Greek Seasoning

1. Preheat oven to 350°F.
2. Line a baking sheet with parchment paper
3. Place almonds on baking sheet
4. Drizzle olive oil over almonds, toss with hands to coat each almond with oil
5. Bake in preheated oven for 10 minutes
6. Remove from oven – pour almonds into small bowl
7. Sprinkle with Greek seasoning
8. Use spatula to toss the warm nuts to coat with seasoning
9. Serve warm or at room temperature.

Air Fried Chickpeas with Greek Seasoning

Chickpeas are trending with health loving foodies as a go-to bean for their high fiber, high protein, availability. I always keep1 or 2 cans on hand for a quick meal or a simple snack of hummus. When reduced to a viscous liquid, the chickpea liquid, aquafaba (bean water), is also treasured. It can replace egg whites to make a fluffy méringue and has many other uses in baking. There are blogs and Facebook pages dedicated to aquafaba. But I will share my amazing adventures with aquafaba another time. This recipe is about crispy, crunchy, tangy, tasty, good for you, chickpeas to snack on.

I try to be mindful of the temptation to buy faddy gadgets that just take up space. But I do love kitchen tools that help me make healthy, plant-based recipes. I've read about the pros and cons of air-fryers for many months – so I finally bought a refurbished Philips fryer to check it out for myself. So far, I've learned that it makes very impressive air-fried chickpeas. I admit I'm still a novice looking forward to tasty experiences ahead.

Ingredients

- 15-ounce can chickpeas – drained but not rinsed
- 4 teaspoons olive oil – divided
- 3 teaspoons homemade "Greek Seasoning Blend" on page 142
- ¼ teaspoon unrefined sea salt
- 2-tablespoons fresh lemon juice

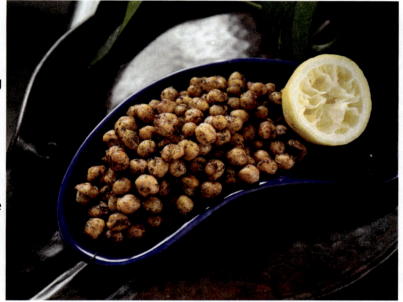

Directions for Air Frying

1. Drain chickpeas but don't rinse – the liquid that remains on the beans will help the spice blend to adhere to the chickpeas.
2. In small bowl, toss the chickpeas with 2 teaspoons of olive oil.
3. Air fry at 400°F for 10 minutes.
4. While chickpeas are frying, whisk together remaining 2 teaspoons of olive oil, 2 tablespoons of lemon juice and 3 teaspoons Greek Seasoning Blend in small bowl.
5. Transfer the cooked chickpeas to small bowl – stir to coat them with dressing
6. Return chickpeas to air fryer and cook for another 10 minutes at 325°F.
7. Serve immediately or store after completely cooled in airtight container.
8. These air-fried chickpeas make a crunchy, lemony snack – they're also interesting to use as croutons on a salad or in a wrap or sandwich – for added texture and flavor.

Oven Roasted Chickpeas with Greek Seasoning

Directions for Oven Roasting

If you don't have an air fryer you could oven roast the chickpeas.

1. Preheat oven to 375° F.
2. Drain chickpeas well but do not rinse.
3. Place chickpeas on a parchment lined baking sheet.
4. Drizzle with 1 tablespoon olive oil and 2 tablespoon lemon juice, and Greek Seasoning Blend - stir to coat chickpeas.
5. Sprinkle with ¼ teaspoon sea salt
6. Place in oven, cook for 15 to 30 minutes, stirring every 5 minutes or so, until golden brown and as crispy to your desired taste.

Almond Coconut Cream

I don't add sweetener or flavoring to my cream, because my husband likes it plain for his coffee.

Ingredients

- 1 cup whole almonds (most of the almond's nutrition is in the skin, so leave it on)
- 2 cups spring or filtered water
- 13.6 ounce can whole fat coconut milk or light coconut milk for less fat - at room temperature –
- Pinch of unrefined sea salt
- Optional: vanilla, cinnamon, sweetener such as dates, maple syrup or agave.

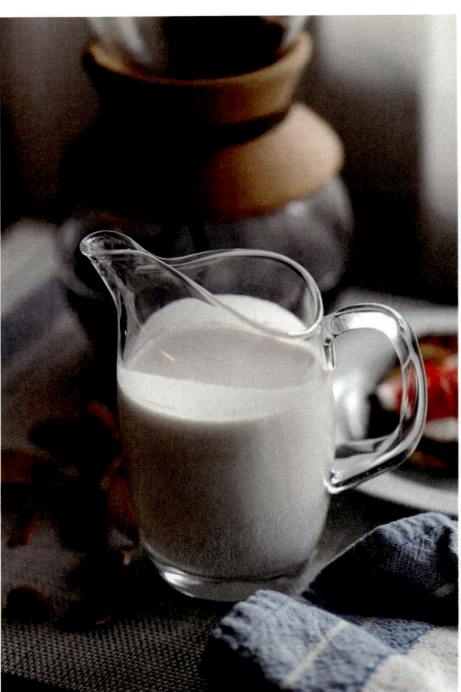

Directions

1. Soak almonds in glass jar, covered with water overnight in the fridge.
2. Drain and rinse almonds.
3. Place almonds in blender with 2 cups of fresh water and blitz on high for a full minute.
4. Pour the milk into a nut milk bag placed over a pitcher or medium size bowl. Gently squeeze the bag to strain the milk from the pulp.
5. Return the strained almond milk to the blender – remove the almond pulp and save for other uses.
6. Shake the can of coconut milk well and add it to the blender with the almond milk, pinch of salt, and sweetener of choice if using.
7. Blitz on medium for 30 seconds to blend the milks together.
8. Transfer the cream to a glass jar with lid and store in refrigerator for up to 5 days.
9. Use creamer in coffee, tea, on oatmeal, cereal, in chia pudding, etc.
10. If cream separates or small coconut fat balls form, just give the jar a good shake to restore a smooth consistency.

Thanks to Thomas at "Full of Plants" blog for the creamer inspiration.

Almond Pulp Cookies

Makes approximately 10 cookies.

Greece, like many Middle Eastern countries, have a thing for almonds. They use them in drinks, candies, preserves, cookies, cakes, etc.. Almonds are placed in high esteem especially when it comes to making sweets. So I have genetically acquired guilt when it comes to discarding leftover almond pulp from making almond milk or almond cream.

Almond cookies are supremely popular in Tarpon's Greek community. So I came up with this no fuss, high protein, gluten-free cookie recipe to use leftover almond pulp. But almond pulp has its challenges. Cookies made with fresh pulp attract moister. When making nut milk, take a little time to gently squeeze out as much liquid from the nut pulp as possible. Baking times may also need some tweaking to firm up the cookie. But with patience, you'll have a tasty almond cookie with a crunchy crust and soft inside.

The cookies tastes better after 1 or 2 days in the fridge. But needs to be reheated for 10-15 minutes in a 325°F oven to remove moisture and refresh their crispy crust.

Ingredients

- Leftover almond pulp from a recipe of "Almond Coconut Cream" on page 132 or "Almond Cream Syrup" on page 134
- 2 tablespoons flax seeds ground to a powder in coffee grinder
- ¼ cup raw cane sugar ground to a powder in coffee grinder
- ¼ teaspoon pure almond or vanilla extract
- ¼ teaspoon cinnamon
- ½ cup sliced almonds
- Tiny pinch of unrefined sea salt
- Optional – confectioners' sugar

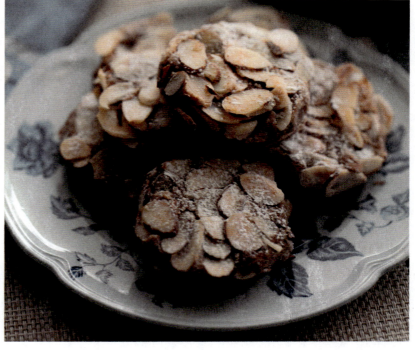

Directions

1. Preheat oven to 350° F.
2. Line a baking sheet with parchment paper.
3. In a medium bowl, combine the almond pulp, ground flax seeds, ground cane sugar, almond extract, and cinnamon – mix well with wooden spoon or your hand.
4. Dough will be wet with the texture of paste – let it rest for 15 minutes to allow the ground flax to bind the dough.
5. Using a small cookie scoop or teaspoon, scoop up the dough and roll it into the sliced almonds.
6. Place the cookies onto the parchment lined baking sheet and lightly press with your fingers to flatten them.
7. Bake on center rack of 350° F preheated oven for 25 minutes.
8. After 25 minutes, turn cookies over and bake an addition 10 minutes or longer to firm them up.
9. Remove cookies from oven and cool to room temperature on baking sheet.
10. Optional: sprinkle cool cookies with confectioners' sugar.
11. When completely cooled, store in Ziploc bag in the fridge – they will keep for up to a week.

Almond Cream Syrup

Yields approximately 2 cups of almond cream syrup.

I make my syrup with the almond skins on because most of the health benefits are in the skin.

Ingredients

- 1 cup almonds with skins
- 2 ½ cups spring water or filtered water
- 1 cup sugar
- 1 cinnamon stick
- 3 whole cloves
- 1 teaspoon pure almond extract I like Nielsen-Massey brand

Directions

1. Place the almonds and water in a blender and blitz on high for 1 minute.
2. Place a large piece of fine mesh cheese cloth over a small sauce pan (I cut a 15 x 16 piece) – pour the almond milk into the center of the cloth – pick up the edges of the cheese cloth and twist the top to enclose the nuts.
3. Gently squeeze the cheese cloth to strain the almond milk from the almond pulp.
4. Using your hands, tie the top of the cheese cloth – and set the ball of pulp aside.
5. Add the sugar, cinnamon stick, and cloves to the saucepan with almond milk.
6. Bring the mixture to a boil over medium heat – boil while stirring with a wooden spoon for 1 minute.
7. Add the cheese cloth that contains the almond pulp to the saucepan.
8. Reduce the heat to low and simmer for 5 minutes – stir the syrup and the cheese cloth containing the pulp with wooden spoon so the contents don't burn.
9. Remove the saucepan from the stove – remove the cheese cloth with almond pulp and set aside.
10. Stir the almond extract into the hot almond syrup and cool to room temperature.
11. Remove the cinnamon stick and cloves.
12. Transfer the syrup to a clean, pint-sized jar with a lid and store in the refrigerator for up to 2 weeks.
13. Use the Almond Syrup to make Almond Cream Soda or blend with nondairy yogurt and top with fruit and nuts.

Almond Cream Syrup blended with plant-based yogurt, topped with fruit & nuts.

Dukkah with Hemp

The first I heard of dukkah was when Chef Joanne Weir mentioned it on her PBS cooking show. I wanted to learn more. Wikipedia lists dukkah as an Egyptian Arabic condiment of nuts, herbs, and spices. Dukkah in Arabic means "to pound" - and that's how dukkah is made. A mixture of spices, herbs, and nuts are pounded in a mortar with a pestle then stirred together to create an exotic seasoning. I use pistachios (my father's favorite nut) for my blend—a pinch of cumin and hemp seeds to kick up the nutritional value with a little omega 3. I think my Egyptian great-grandfather would be proud.

Ingredients

- ¼ cup pistachios
- 1 teaspoon black peppercorns
- 1-teaspoon coriander seeds
- 1 teaspoon sesame seeds
- 1 teaspoon black sesame seeds
- ½ teaspoon cumin seeds
- ½ teaspoon fennel seeds
- 1 teaspoon dried mint
- 1 teaspoon dried thyme
- 2 tablespoons hemp-seeds
- ½ teaspoon unrefined sea salt

Directions

1. Using a mortar and pestle or a spice grinder - pound or grind separately the pistachios, peppercorns, coriander seeds, sesame seeds, cumin and fennel seeds.
2. Stir together with dried mint, thyme, hemp seeds and salt – mix until blended.
3. Store in airtight jar. Will keep in refrigerator for 1 month.
4. Serve with olive oil as a dip with fresh bread. Also delicious sprinkled on hard boiled organic, free-range eggs.

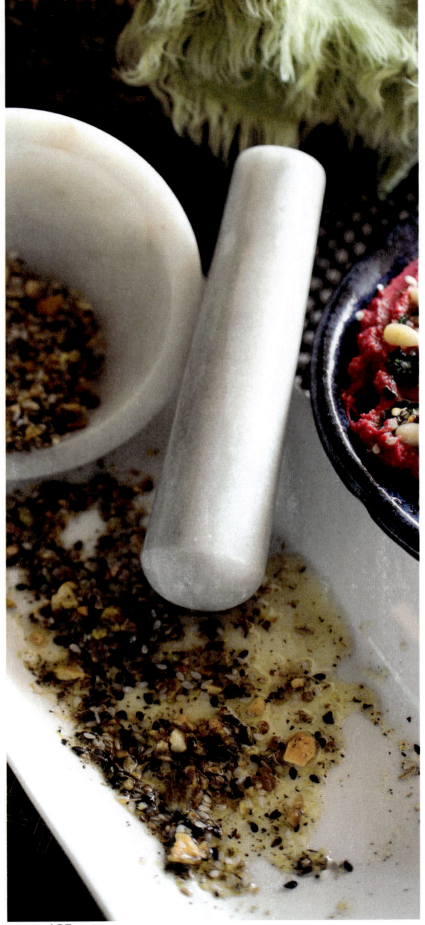

Bread – A Greek Love Affair

"If thou tastest a crust of bread, thou tastest all the stars and all the heavens."

– Robert Browning

My father used to say that a slice of crusty bread fresh from the oven was one of the simplest ways to experience the joy of life. My daughters would tell you their #1 food craving is a humble piece of homemade bread. Some of my most cherished memories are of getting up early on a winter morning to fill the house with the aromas of coffee brewing and bread baking.

When I cooked for the friars' I tried to make a daily small loaf to serve with their meal. I used a bread machine to mix and knead the dough. I would transfer the dough from the machine to an oiled bowl to rise, then baked it off in a hot oven. Like my father, the friars considered bread sacred. If a piece accidentally fell to the ground they would pick it up - raise it to heaven, "Kiss it to God," and consume it.

This is my basic Greek loaf recipe. A preferment and optional beer give it a yeasty flavor. Make the preferment the night before. A preferment is simply water, flour, and yeast that's allowed to ferment overnight. This simple extra step adds character to the loaf. https://en.wikipedia.org/wiki/Preferment.

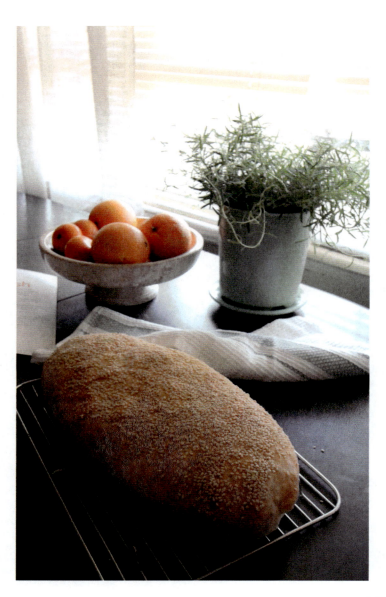

Preferment Ingredients

Plan ahead, make the preferment the night before.

- 1/3-cup spring water
- ½ cup bread flour
- 1-teaspoon instant or rapid rise yeast

Preferment Directions

1. In bowl, blend the water, flour and yeast together with a wooden spoon.
2. Cover the bowl with plastic wrap and allow to ferment at room temperature overnight.

Bread Ingredients

1. 4 cups bread flour – plus a little more if needed
2. 3 teaspoons instant or rapid rise yeast
3. 1 teaspoon unrefined sea salt
4. 1 recipe Preferment
5. 2 tablespoons olive oil
6. 1 ½ cups water or beer - Greek Mythos or Budweiser
7. Optional – 2 tablespoons sesame seeds
8. Coarse cornmeal for baking

Directions

1. In mixing bowl, whisk together the bread flour, instant yeast, and salt.
2. Place pre-ferment, olive oil, and beer into mixing bowl with flour. Place dough hook on mixer.
3. Start mixer on low speed and mix until a dough starts to form, scraping down sides as needed.
4. Increase speed to medium low and knead for 15 to 20 minutes, or until dough is smooth and clears the sides of the bowl.
5. Transfer the dough to a lightly oiled medium bowl – cover tightly with plastic wrap and let it rise for 1 hour or until doubled in bulk.
6. Gently press the air out of dough, transfer to a lightly floured counter.
7. Knead a few times then divide into 2 portions.
8. Shape and knead into 2 loaves – place seam side down on baking sheet lined with parchment paper sprinkled with coarse corn meal.
9. Brush each loaf with water and sprinkle with 1 tablespoon of sesame seeds.
10. Loosely cover the loaves with a kitchen towel and allow to rise another 45 minutes or until they have doubled.
11. Position oven rack in lower middle of oven.
12. Preheat oven to 450° F.
13. Bake the loaves in 450° preheated oven for 25 to 35 minutes or until golden and hollow when tapped.
14. Cool complete on rack before serving
15. Serve with olive oil and Greek spice blend for dipping, spoon sweets, and/or with other mezzes.
16. Note: Bread can be kneaded in the bowl of a bread machine or by hand until smooth and elastic. After kneading, proceed with the recipe and listed.

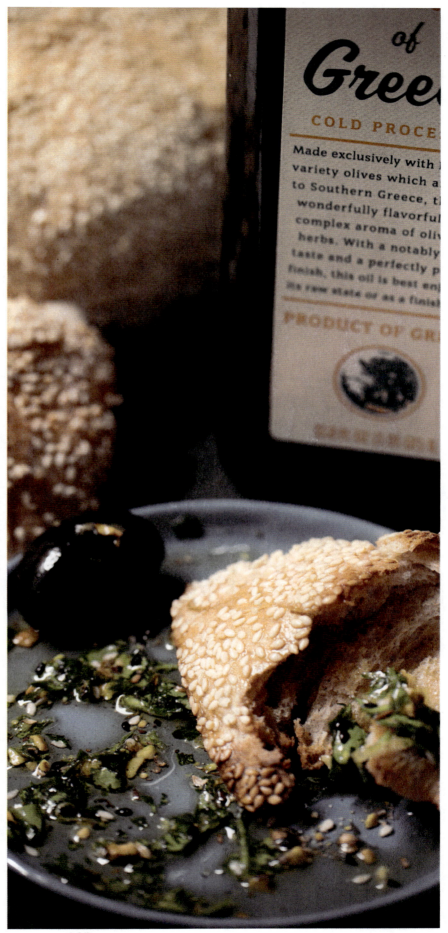

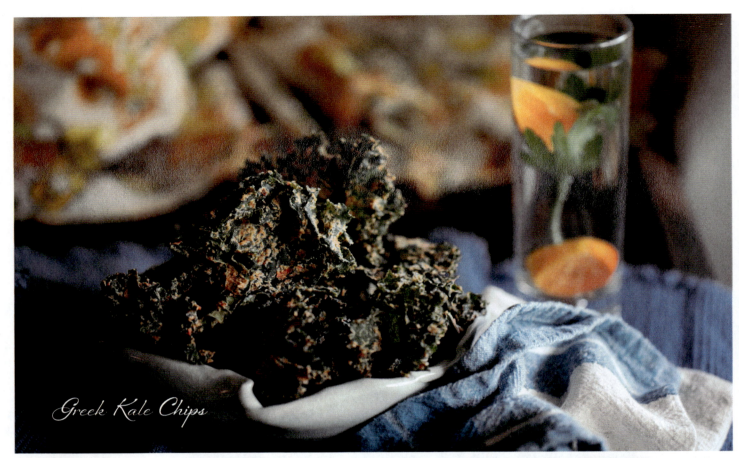
Greek Kale Chips

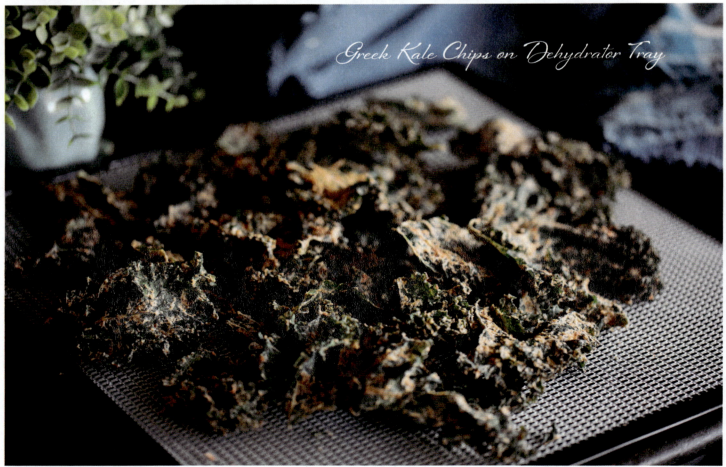
Greek Kale Chips on Dehydrator Tray

Greek Kale Chips

Kale chips make an interesting, yummy, superfood snack, and I love to serve them for mezze gatherings. They are trendy, super healthy, and make an exceptionally delicious alternative to potato chips. Kale chips can be purchased from health food stores but be prepared to pay big bucks for a small bag. I have a 9-tray Excalibur Dehydrator that makes crispy, off the charts delicious, Greek seasoned chips. But this recipe can also be baked in the oven.

In addition to serving as a mezze, kale chips makes a fantastic treat for Superbowl or as a special treat to share at work.

I've made this recipe with Dino and curly kale. Curly kale definitely makes the best chips.

Ingredients Seasoning Mix

- 1 bunch curly kale, stems removed, washed, dried, and leaves torn into large pieces.
- 1 cup cashews soaked at least 3 hours in spring water or overnight.
- 1 small red bell pepper seeded and chopped
- 1 tablespoon "Greek Seasoning Blend" on page 142
- 1 tablespoon nutritional yeast
- 1 tablespoon fresh lemon juice
- ½ teaspoon unrefined sea salt

Directions Seasoning Mixture

- Drain and rinse cashews, and place in blender or mini-food processor with red bell pepper, seasoning blend, nutritional yeast, lemon juice, and salt.
- Pulse until creamy scraping down sides as needed.

Dehydrated Kale Chips

1. Place leaves in large bowl – spoon creamy seasoning mixture onto leaves, and gently toss using hands to coat each leaf with mixture.
2. Place on dehydrator tray(s) in single layer.
3. Dehydrate at 115° F for 3 to 5 hours – check after 2 hours.
4. Serve at room temperature and watch them disappear!
5. Best if served the same day but will keep a day or two in a tightly sealed Ziploc bag.

Oven Baked Kale Chips

1. Preheat oven to 300° F
2. Wash and dry kale.
3. Remove stems and tear leaves into large pieces.
4. Place leaves in large bowl with seasoning mixture – gently toss to coat each leaf with mixture.
5. Line baking sheet with parchment paper.
6. Place leaves in a single layer on baking pan.
7. Bake in preheated oven for 20 to 25 minutes, rotating the pan half way through cooking.
8. Cool to room temperature.
9. Best if served the same day.

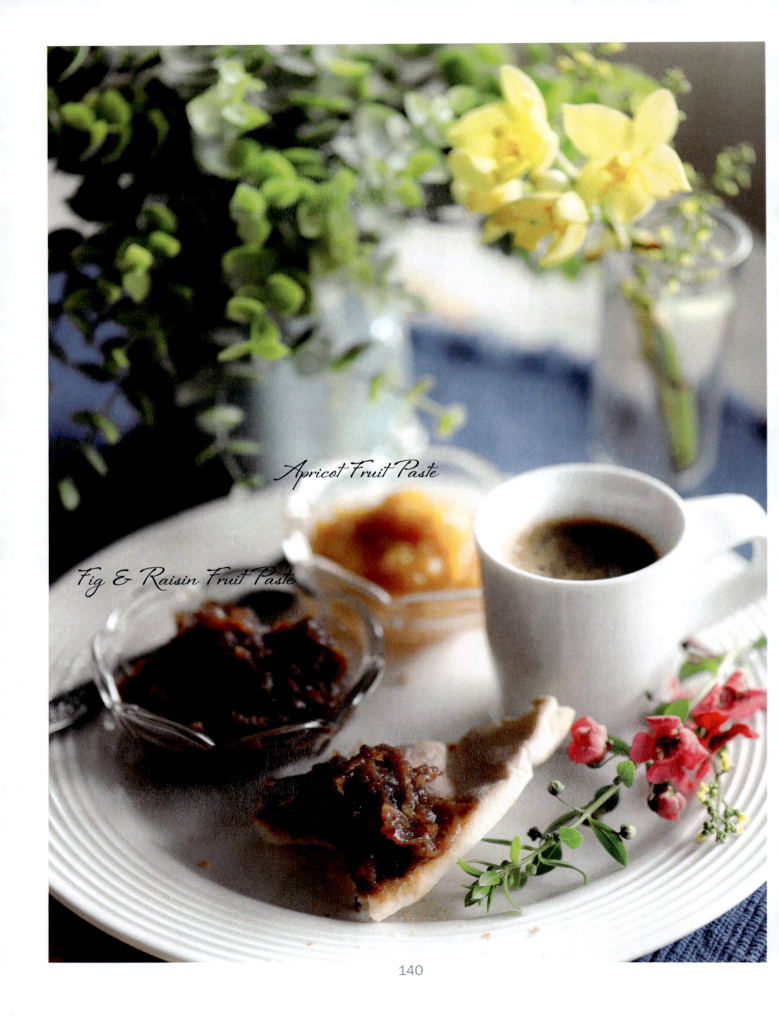

Fig & Raisin Fruit Paste with Anise & Cinnamon

Makes 1/2 cup of paste.

My mother made fruit pastes. Her method was to slow cook dried fruits with water and lots of white sugar for an hour or longer. Then she used the paste to make cookies or turnovers. I learned from Rouxbe cooking school that fruit pastes can also be used as full-flavored, whole food sweeteners for smoothies, dressings, etc. I love fruit paste on my toast and swirled in steel-cut oatmeal. It makes a rich and flavorful mezze.

Rouxbe uses a no-cook method and no added sugar procedure that is much more simple and just as yummy as my mother's. I use their technique to make my fruit pastes but infuse them with flavors from my Greek American kitchen.

Ingredients

- 8 Calimyrna figs stems removed
- 2 tablespoons raisins
- ½ teaspoon anise seeds
- ¼ teaspoon ground cinnamon
- 1 cup spring or filtered water

Directions

1. Place the figs, raisins, anise seeds, and cinnamon in a small bowl – cover with the water.
2. Cover and refrigerate for 4 hours.
3. Transfer to a blender and pulse until smooth.
4. If too thick, add small amounts of water to thin consistency - should be paste-like, not runny.
5. Serve with warm pita, toasted Greek bread, swirl in oatmeal on top of plant yogurt – or use your own imagination.

Apricot or Date Paste

Replace figs and raisins with 1/2 cup dried apricots or seeded dates. Omit the anise seeds and follow directions as for Fig & Raisin Paste.

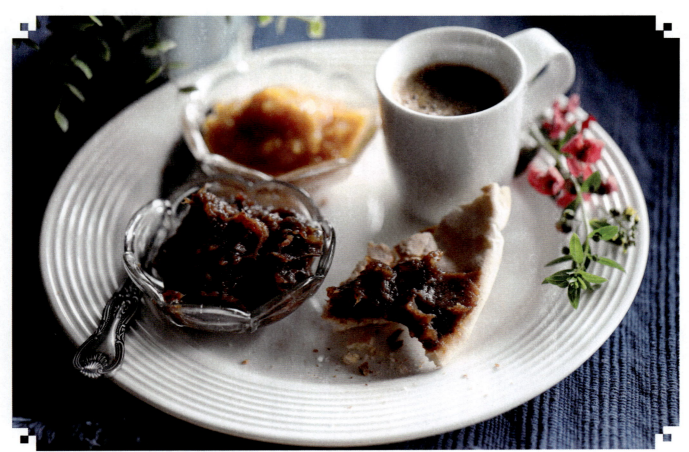

Greek Seasoning Blend

If you like commercial Greek seasoning – you'll love our family's Greek seasoning blend! It makes a delicious herby seasoning for salad dressings; it's fantastic with olive oil for dipping, stir it into vegan mayo and sour cream for a phenomenal veggie dip, or use it for a tasty sprinkle on top of hummus and/or roasted veggies. It's a perfect flavoring for plant-based Greek meatloaf, and it makes an exquisite gourmet gift. Hope you'll give it a try!

Ingredients

- 2-tablespoons dried oregano
- 1-tablespoon black pepper
- 1-tablespoon dried basil
- 1-tablespoon dried dill
- 1-tablespoon dried mint
- 1-tablespoon dried onion flakes
- 1 tablespoon dried parsley (dried)
- 1-tablespoon dried rosemary
- 2-teaspoons dried marjoram
- 2 teaspoons dried thyme
- 1-teaspoon dried garlic granules

Directions

1. Place all ingredients in coffee or spice grinder and pulse to blend.
2. Alternatively, combine all ingredients in small bowl —whisk to blend.
3. Store in clean glass container/jar with lid.
4. Keep in a cool dark place.
5. Will keep for 6 months.

Gremolata

Gremolata adds superfood nutrients, flavor, and a wow factor to your mezzes. I love it on my plant-based keftedes, chickpeas, Greek lemon potatoes, lentil salad, soups, etc.

Variations: use dandelion greens, parsley, cilantro, power greens, or your favorite green.

Ingredients

- 1 small bunch(approximately 1 cup) of your choice of greens –
- 1 garlic clove minced
- 1 tablespoon olive oil
- 2 teaspoons fresh lemon juice
- 1/8 teaspoon salt
- Lemon zest from 1 organic lemon

Directions

1. Place all ingredients, except for lemon zest, in bowl of small food processor.
2. Pulse until chopped and blended.
3. Spoon chopped gremolata into serving bowl and stir in lemon zest.
4. Gremolata will keep covered in fridge for about 5 days.

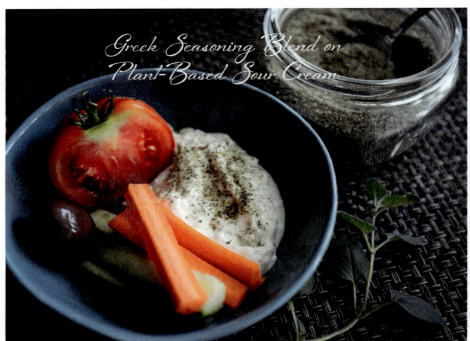

Grilled Greek Toasts

1. 1/2-inch slices of Greek, French, or Italian bread.
2. Place bread slices on hot grill and cover.
3. Grill 2 to 3 minutes or until bread is toasted and grill marks appear.
4. Turn slices over and grill the other side - for 2 to 3 minutes with grill covered.
5. Once grill marks appear, remove and serve with mezzes.

Grilled Pita Breads

1. 1 or more pita or naan breads.
2. Place pita or naan on hot grill and cover.
3. Grill 2 to 3 minutes or until bread is lightly toasted with grill marks.
4. Turn pita or naan over and grill the other side for 2 to 3 minutes with grill covered.
5. Once grill marks appear, remove and serve with mezzes.

Balsamic Cinnamon Syrup

My daughter and son-in-law love to try out trendy cafes. She often tells me how disappointed she is at their desserts. She blames it on the deliciousness of my Balsamic Cinnamon Syrup.

It's simple to make for the amount of "mmm" it provides. Balsamic vinegar reduction infused with cinnamon makes a richly flavored drizzle. It adds a depth of deliciousness that will impress.

I love to use it as a sweetener for my raw Spoon Sweets and Roasted Fruits. It's also yummy on top of nondairy ice cream, yogurt, fruit salads, or drizzled on a slice of cake.

Ingredients

- 1 cup organic balsamic vinegar
- 3 tablespoons agave nectar
- 1 cinnamon stick

Directions

1. Combine the vinegar, agave, and cinnamon stick in small saucepan.
2. Bring to a boil over medium heat stirring often.
3. Reduce heat to allow a low simmer uncovered and cook until reduced by half – about 10 minutes.
4. Syrup should coat the back of a spoon.
5. Remove pot from stove and cool to room temperature with cinnamon stick remaining in syrup.
6. Store covered in refrigerator – will keep for a couple of weeks.

Mint & Cinnamon Simple Syrup

Mint is one of the mystery ingredients that gives Greek cooking its essence. My yia yia had a patch of spearmint that grew wild in her side yard. She always had a few bunches bundled, along with other herbs, hanging on her kitchen wall to dry. They were placed right next to a small, iconic painting of a saint who looked down on me with a disapproving stare.

I love to explore my ancestors' flavors, and mint is one of the herbs at the top of my list. Just like yia yia, I use it for sweet and savory recipes. I also made peace with the icon – who is Saint Nicholas. Now he hangs out with me on my kitchen wall. I believe the years and possibly my joy of cooking have softened him. Depending on the day, and the recipe, sometimes he even shoots me a little smile.

Ingredients

- 1 cup dry white wine (La Crema chardonnay is plant-based) or use spring or filtered water
- 1 cup raw cane sugar
- 1 cinnamon stick
- 1 small bunch fresh mint

Directions

1. Heat wine (or water), cinnamon, and sugar in small saucepan over medium heat.
2. Bring to a boil – boil for 3 minutes or until sugar is fully dissolved.
3. Remove from saucepan with syrup from heat.
4. Cook to room temperature - remove mint & cinnamon stick
5. Pull mint leaves from the stems – tear and crush the leaves with your hands, and drop them into the hot syrup – stir to submerge the leaves in the syrup - cont. on next page

Mint & Cinnamon Simple Syrup cont.

6. Cool to room temperature, strain the syrup, and transfer to a glass jar with lid.
7. Store in refrigerator for up to a month.

Use this syrup to sweeten iced tea, lemonade, or other cold beverages. It's yummy on fruit – especially honey dew melon and berries.

Orange Spiced Wine Syrup

Ingredients

- 1 cup evaporated cane sugar
- 3/4 cup dry white wine, like La Crema Chardonnay
- Juice from 1 organic orange
- Rind from 1 organic orange
- 1 cinnamon stick
- 1-teaspoon fresh lemon juice

Directions

1. Combine cane sugar, wine, juice, orange peel, and cinnamon stick in a small saucepan.
2. Bring to a boil over medium-high heat and boil for 3 minutes.
3. Reduce heat to simmer and simmer uncovered for 10 minutes.
4. Remove from heat and cool to room temperature with orange peel and cinnamon stick remaining in syrup.
5. Stir fresh lemon juice into cooled syrup.

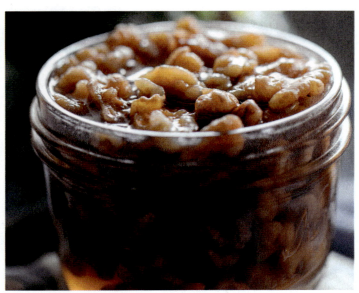

Spiced Wine Syrup

Ingredients

- 1-cup cane sugar
- 1 cup white wine like La Crema Chardonnay
- Rind of 1 organic lemon
- 2 cinnamon sticks
- 2 whole cloves
- 1-teaspoon fresh lemon juice

Directions

1. Combine sugar, wine, rind, cinnamon stick, and cloves, in small saucepan.
2. Bring to boil over medium high heat and boil for 3 minutes.
3. Reduce heat and simmer syrup uncovered for 10 minutes.
4. Remove from heat, stir in lemon juice, and cool with spices.
5. Once cool, remove spices and lemon rind.
6. Spoon cooled syrup onto hot baklava, hot cake, fruit salad, or use in other recipes as directed.

Wet Walnuts in Spiced Wine Syrup

Yields 1 half pint.

Ingredients

- ½ pint jar
- Enough walnuts or pistachios to fill a half pint jar

Directions

1. Fill a clean glass Mason jar with walnuts or unsalted pistachios.
2. Pour enough cool Spiced Syrup over the nuts to cover them.
3. Cover the jar with a lid and store in the refrigerator for up to 2 weeks.
4. Serve over plant-based ice cream, yogurt, on oatmeal, in fruit salads, etc.

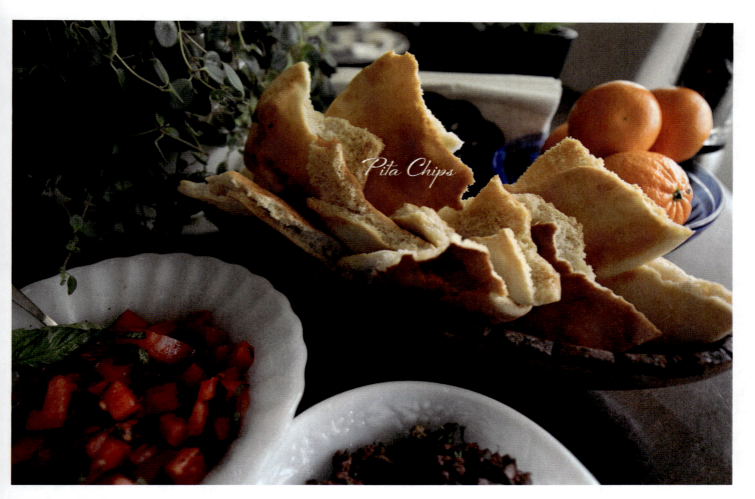

Pita Chips

Pita breads are hollow in the center. When I make pita chips, I open the pita breads then cut them into triangles or hand tear them into pieces to make chips. You can also make chips with flatbread or naan. But these breads are not hollow, so you'll need to increase the baking time by 5 minutes or more to ensure they're cooked through.

Ingredients

- Preheat oven to 400°F
- 2 pita breads opened, each round cut or torn into 8 pieces. You should have 16 pieces per pita.
- 2 tablespoons olive oil
- 5 grinds fresh pepper from mill
- Sprinkles of unrefined sea salt

Directions

1. Using pastry brush, lightly brush pita pieces with olive oil on both sides
2. Sprinkle lightly with sea salt and pepper
3. Bake on parchment lined baking sheet on center rack of oven for 15 to 20 minutes, turning once or twice during cooking. Pita chips should be light golden brown.
4. Serve at room temperature with hummus, tzatziki, Greek Guac, bruschetta, etc..

Prosphoro - Greek Offering Bread

Makes 2 large and 6 small loaves.

My mother was Irish and Methodist. My father was Greek Orthodox. We were baptized Methodist and mostly went to the Methodist Church. But my father loved the Greek Church – and so on special occasions he would sneak my sister and me into a Greek Mass. I found it deeply enchanting and beautiful. I remember staring in wonder at the iconic artwork painted on the walls and ceiling, I was spellbound by the Greek priest's chants, and intoxicated by the peculiar perfume of the incense.

Another fascination I have with the Greek Church is a custom that began with the early Christians. Women bring loaves of home baked bread that is blessed by the priest then becomes the "prosphoro" or the Communion Bread - the Bread of Life. These offering breads are stamped with a religious seal "sfraýitha" that can be purchased from a Greek monastery or from online specialty stores.

To be clear, this bread does not become the Offering Bread or Eucharist without a priest's blessing. But I love to teach my grandchildren about their Greek roots by creating a spiritual atmosphere in my home, which includes making these beautiful loaves. I light candles and play chant to invite the Spirit of Love to our gathering - then we enjoy the loaves usually smeared with butter and Spoon Sweets.

Ingredients

- You will need a prosphoro stamp, which can be purchased from Amazon or a Greek Monastery (see source page for details)
- 1-½ cups warm water
- 1-teaspoon sea salt
- 3 teaspoons instant yeast
- 4 cups unbleached bread flour – plus a little more if needed

Directions

1. Set bread machine to knead for 20 minutes - or knead by hand.
2. Add water, salt, yeast, and flour to bread machine bowl or to a large mixing bowl if not using bread machine.
3. Turn bread machine on - knead for 20 minutes – add flour a little at a time but only if needed, or hand knead till smooth and elastic
4. Remove the dough from the machine
5. Place dough in a bowl – cover with a damp dish towel and let it rise for 1 to 1-1/2 hours or until doubled in bulk
6. Press air out of dough
7. Cut dough into 2 pieces – cut one piece into 2 and the second piece into 6 smaller pieces.
8. Dust clean counter-top with flour and roll all pieces into balls then with hands stretch and pull each ball into a round slab – place on parchment lined baking sheet making sure to leave plenty of space between each to allow for rising and stamping - cover with damp dish towel, and allow to rise for 45-60 minutes or until doubled.
9. Preheat oven to 400°F
10. Place 1 large dough round on top of the second large dough round.
11. Using a pastry brush, brush the large side of bread stamp with flour and press it onto the top bread round.
12. Using large side of stamp, press design deeply on to the top of the double loaf
13. Flip stamp to small design - dust with flour and stamp the remaining 6 small loaves.
14. Bake in preheated oven for 30 to 40 minutes or until golden brown
15. Remove and cool on rack
16. Say a prayer of thanksgiving for how beautiful your loaves look and how wonderful your kitchen smells
17. Pass the plant butter or olive oil .

Amen!

Prosphora – Greek Offering Breads

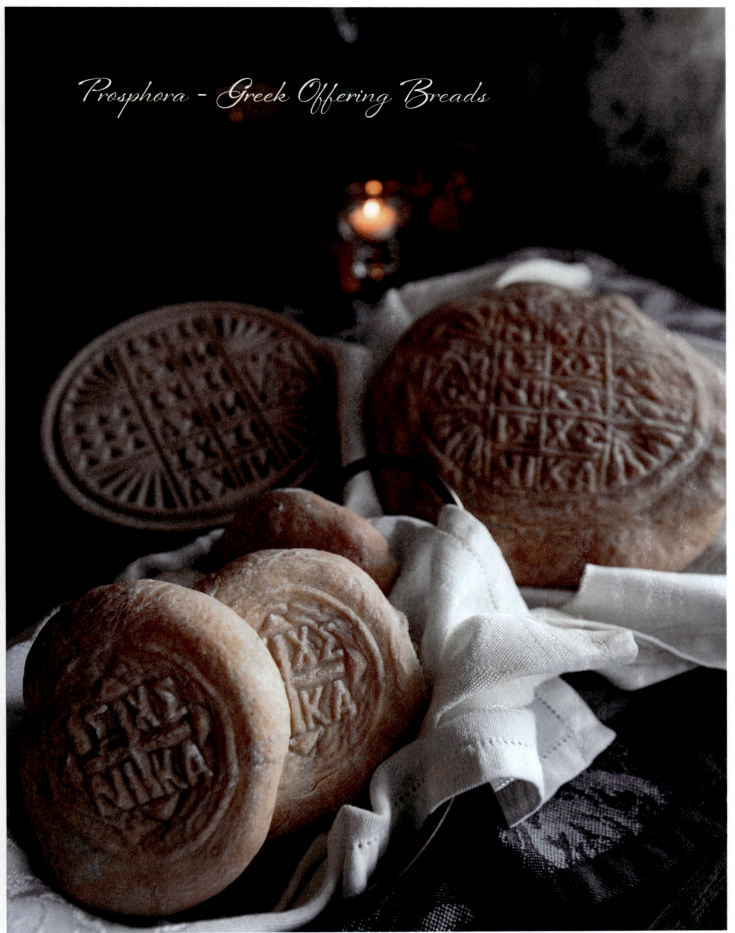

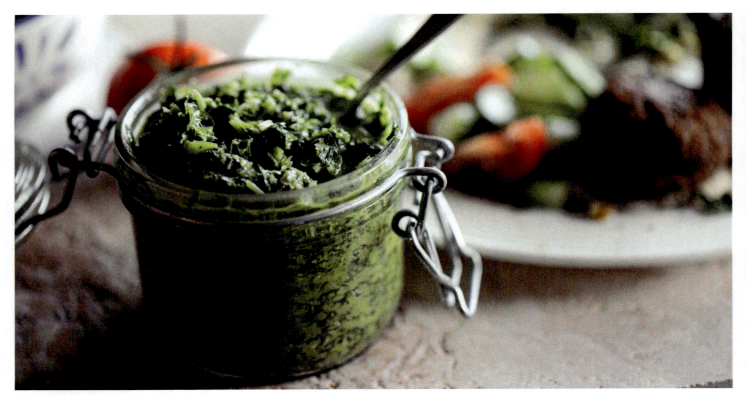

Schug

A spicy hot Mediterranean condiment. This little jar of fresh green goodness wakes up any recipe. It's so yummy you may (like me) become addicted. Serve it with roasted veggies, falafel, on hummus, in soups or as a simple dip for pita bread. If you like more heat, leave the seeds in the jalapenos – but beware - this condiment is already pretty hot.

Ingredients

- 2 jalapeño peppers - remove stem, veins, and seeds
- 1 bunch fresh cilantro
- 1 bunch curly or flat Italian parsley
- 6 garlic cloves, finely minced
- ½ teaspoon unrefined sea salt
- ¼ teaspoon ground coriander
- 1/8 teaspoon ground cumin
- 3 or 4 grinds fresh milled pepper
- 2 tablespoons quality olive oil
- 1 tablespoon fresh lemon juice

Spicy!

Directions

1. Remove seeds and veins from jalapenos and coarsely chop.
2. Remove 1 or 2 inches of stems from the cilantro and parsley, leave remaining stems and leaves and coarsely chop.
3. Add all ingredients to food processor bowl fitted with steel blade and pulse until coarsely chopped and blended.
4. Store in glass jar for 5 days to 1 week.

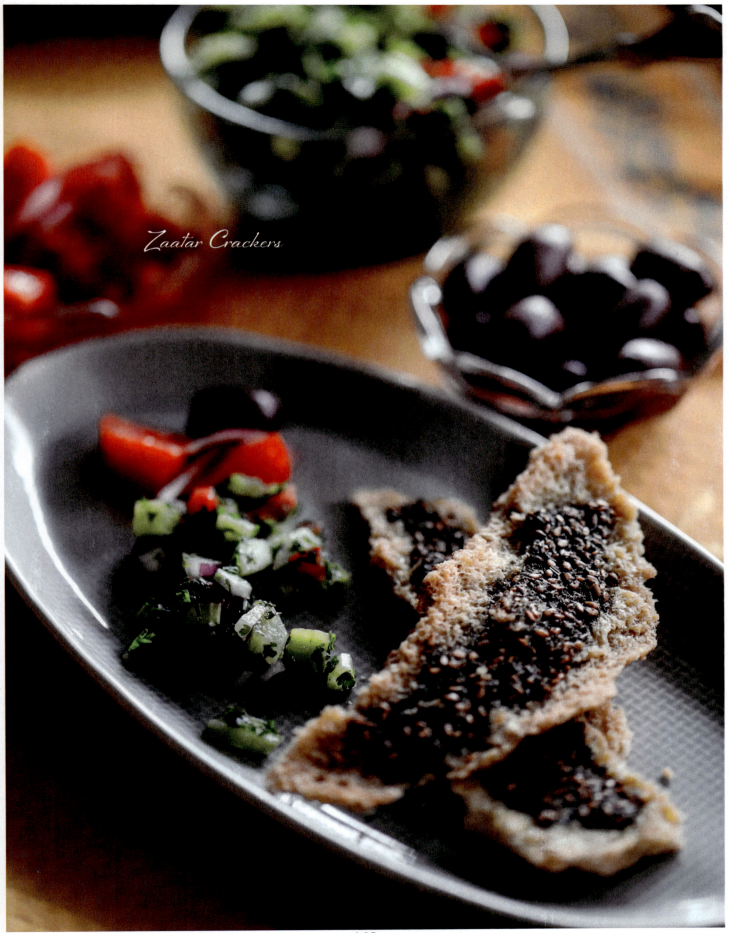
Zaatar Crackers

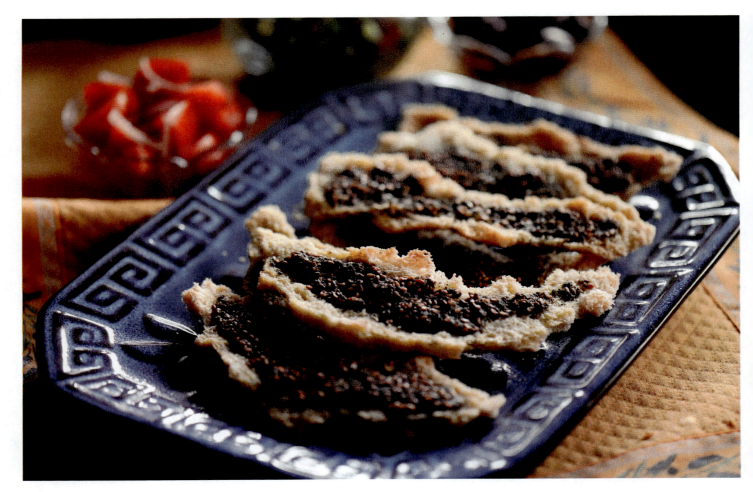

Zaatar Crackers Recipe

These free form crackers are uniquely delicious and make an interesting mezze.

Ingredients

- 2 pita rounds (I used 8-inch pitas)
- Unrefined sea salt
- 3 tablespoons olive oil
- 2 tablespoons zaatar herb blend

Directions

1. Preheat oven to 375° F.
2. In a small bowl, stir the olive oil and zaatar together to blend – set aside.
3. Using your hands, tear the pita rounds open, then tear each round into free-form strips.
4. Place pita strips onto parchment lined baking sheet and lightly sprinkle with salt.
5. Bake on center rack of preheated oven for 5 minutes.
6. Remove from oven and lightly spoon a little of the zaatar mixture down the center of each strip.
7. Return the strips to the oven and bake for another 3 to 4 minutes, or until crackers turn golden brown on the edges.
8. Remove from the oven and cool completely before serving.
9. Store in Ziploc bag, will keep a couple of days.

Greek-ish Pantry

This is a list of pantry staples I like to keep on hand. I buy most of my dried herbs, beans, and grains from the bulk section of health food stores. The ingredients are organic, less expensive, and buying in bulk helps the planet by reducing excessive packaging waste. Buying in small amounts also ensures my ingredients are fresh.

Even our cats know the difference between bulk, organic catnip and prepackaged catnip from department stores. They go crazy from the moment I walk through the front door with a small baggie of "nip." They circle me and nudge my legs, and won't leave me alone till I give them a little pinch of herby catmint, aka catnip. I love seeing them so happy.

Greek Spice List

I shop at Mediterranean markets for the herbs and spices I use most commonly such as oregano, mint, zaatar and sumac. But other herbs and spices I buy from the bulk sections of local health food stores and I buy small amounts. This makes it more economical so I can afford organic, it's less wasteful and it ensures the freshest possible ingredients for my recipes.

ALLSPICE

A small hard berry that tastes like all the spices.

ANISE SEEDS

Anise seeds are used to flavor ouzo. I love them simmered and used to flavor bread or pounded with mortar and pestle for preserves and jams. I purchase anise seeds from a Mediterranean market – where I find the best value.

BLACK & WHITE PEPPERCORNS

My first cooking instructor insisted we grind our own peppercorns for freshness and flavor - and I've been faithful to that practice. I purchase peppercorns from Ross, Marshall's and HomeGoods stores.

CARDAMOM

Aromatic seeds that come from pods. Ground to use in sweets and to flavor Greek, Turkish or Arabic coffee.

CINNAMON

Possibly the most commonly used spice in Greek cooking. Used in sweet and savory recipes.

CLOVES

Cloves are very aromatic – a little goes a long way. Just like cinnamon, cloves are used in sweet and savory recipes.

MAHLEPI SEEDS

The tiny pits from wild cherries that grow in the Mediterranean and Middle East. It's best to use only whole seeds – ground seeds become rancid and quickly lose their flavor. Store seeds in freezer to maintain their freshness. They are used to flavor sweets, special syrups, Greek holiday breads, and cakes.

NIGELLA SEEDS

I substitute black sesame seeds. They are most commonly used to sprinkle on breads.

SEA SALT

I use Redmond Ancient Fine Grains – a high quality unfiltered, natural sea salt. I also love Maldon Salt as a finishing salt.

Greek Herbs List

BASIL

Fresh and dried basil in savory recipes.

BAY LEAF

Dried leaves used as a flavoring for soups, stews and sauces. The leaf can cause intestinal problems so should be used whole then discarded before serving.

DILL

Fresh and dried used for savory recipes.

GARLIC

Mostly fresh garlic. Sliced, minced or mashed for savory recipes and salad dressings.

GREEK OREGANO

Very common herb in Greek cooking, like mint, I buy it in 1-pound packages from the Mediterranean market, Ziyad brand reminds me most of the oregano used in my family's kitchen. I personally do not care for fresh oregano, so I only use dried.

MARJORAM

Similar to oregano, used in savory recipes.

MINT

Fresh mint and dried mint are commonly used in Greek recipes. Mint is also brewed to make a refreshing hot or cold tea. I purchase dried mint by the pound from a local Mediterranean market, Sadaf brand.

SAGE

A savory leafy herb used fresh and/or dried for savory recipes and steeped to make tea.

SUMAC

Sumac is a berry found in regions of the Mediterranean. It's ground, like pepper, into a fine powder. It has a very bold, tart, lemony flavor. It can be found in large grocery store chains or from Amazon or Frontier Co-op Spice Co.

THYME
Fresh and dried are both used in Greek cooking. I prefer fresh thyme in my recipes – but use dried in my Greek Spice Blend.

ZAATAR
Middle Eastern Seasoning Blend. I like green zaatar - look for "green" zaatar for a flavorful blend. Available from Amazon or Frontier Co-op Spice Company.

Shopping

BEER:
Mythos Greek Beer or Budweiser are listed as plant-based friendly on Barnivore website.

BRIKI GREEK COFFEE POT:
Available from Amazon, Etsy, and Mediterranean markets.

COCONUT MILK:
Thai Kitchen Organic Unsweetened Coconut Milk

EXTRACTS:
Nielsen-Massey Pure Almond Extract. Nielsen-Massey Organic Fairtrade Madagascar Bourbon Pure Vanilla Extract

FETA:
Violife Plant Based Feta available at grocery stores, Whole Foods Market, and health food stores.

GREEK COFFEE:
Loumidis, Papagalos Traditional Greek Coffee or Bravo brand Greek - Coffee. Both available at Mediterranean markets or Amazon. Instant Frappe: Nescafé - may be found at Mediterranean or Middle Eastern markets, and Amazon.

NAMA SHOYU
Nama Shoyu is a raw, unpasteurized soy sauce. May be found at Whole Foods, Amazon, or other health food stores. My favorite brand is Ohsawa Organic Nama Shoyu.

NON-DAIRY BUTTER:
Milkadamia Salted Buttery Spread, Miyoko's European Style Cultured Vegan Butter, and Smart Balance brands.

NON-DAIRY MILK:

I use unsweetened almond milk or soy milk. I also make a rich cream by blending homemade almond milk with canned coconut milk.

NON-DAIRY YOGURT:

I mostly use Kite Hill brand. Silk makes good almond milk yogurt too.

OLIVES:

I buy olives with seeds then remove the pits myself – I find whole olives much more flavorful. I use a mixture of these olives: Castelvetrano, Kalamata Olives, Moroccan or Oil Cured

OLIVE OIL:

First Cold Pressed oils offer the most polyphenols. Extra Light Olive Oil for frying.

PHYLLO:

Athens brand. Comes packaged in 2, 8-ounce rolls of phyllo dough for baklava and spanakopita.

HOLY BREAD STAMP/SEAL:

Bread stamps are sold on Amazon but Monastiriaka.gr, a Greek Monastery sells high quality bread seals and other items.

SHERRY:

Williams & Humbert Dry Sack Medium Sherry. Vegan and plant-based friendly. Adds depth of flavor to recipes.

SWEETNERS:

100% maple syrup, agave nectar, and raw organic cane sugar.

TEA:

Klio brand for Shepherd's Tea found on Amazon. Lipton Organic Black Tea for various recipes.

WHISKEY:

Ballentine's Finest Scotch Whiskey. Available at most large liquor stores. Barnivore lists it as plant-based and vegan friendly.

WINE:

La Crema Chardonnay dry, buttery, delicious wine. Barnivore lists it as plant-based and vegan friendly. I love to use it in my cooking – it's also yummy to sip.

References

American Holistic Nurses Association, Board Certification: https://www.ahna.org

Barnivore Guide to Plant-Based Wine, Beer, and Liquor. https://www.barnivore.com

Barnard, N. MD Retrieved from PCRM, Physicians Committee for Responsible Medicine: https://www.pcrm.org

Barnard, N. MD. The Exam Room Physicians Committee for Responsible Medicine. Apple Podcast or Spotify.

Beard, James. James Beard Foundation - https://www.jamesbeard.org.

Campbell, T. C. MD (2005). The China Study. United States: BenBella Books.

Capuchin Franciscans Providence of the Sacred Stigmat of St. Francis. Retrieved from https://capuchinfriars.org. Fr. Remo DiSalvatore, OFM Cap. Provincial Minister.

City of Tarpon Springs Website. (n.d.). Retrieved from City Government Website: https://www.ctsfl.us

Cousins, Gabriel MD. (2000). Conscious Eating and (2005) Spiritual Nutrition, Berkeley: North Atlantic Books. Website: http://treeoflifecenterus.com

Davis, G. M. (2015). Proteinaholic: How Our Obsession with Meat is Killing Us and What We Can Do About It. New York: HarperOne.

Deryn. Running on Real Food - Blog. Retrieved from https://runningonrealfood.com

Esselstyn, R. (2009, 2017). Engine 2 Diet. New York: Grand Central Publishing.

Fermentation Fundamentals. Chef Frank Giglio, Farm & Forage Kitchen. http://farmandforagekitchen.com/about

Fuhrman, J. MD (2020). Eat For Life. New York: HarperOne.

Greger, M. MD (2015). How Not to Die. New York: Flatiron Books.

Greger, M. MD. Nutrition Facts website Retrieved from https://nutritionfacts.org

Harvard Health Letter, (2013). Healthier Oils Makes Fried Food Safer.

Harvard School of Public Health, TH Chan, https://www.hsph.harvard.edu

Kenney, M. (n.d.). Matthew Kenney Culinary Academy. Retrieved from https://www.matthewkenneycuisine.com/food-future-institute

Kochilas, D. Greek Food for Life. Retrieved from https://www.dianekochilas.com/blog/

Love, E. (n.d.). BodyMind Institute. Retrieved from Elaina Love Raw Food Certification: https://bodymindinstitute.com/raw-chef-certification/

Madison, D. (2011). The New Vegetarian Cooking for Everyone. Berkeley: Ten Speed Press.

Minaki, P. (n.d.). Kalofagas Greek Food and Beyond. Retrieved from https://www.kalofagas.ca

Monastiriaka - Mount Athos. (n.d.). Retrieved from Monastic Products: https://www.monastiriaka.gr/en/

Moskowitz, I. and Romero, Terry (2017). Veganomicon. New York: Da Capo Life Long Books.

National Health Association Publisher of Health Science Magazine. https://www.healthscience.org/about/about-nha

Palmer, S. a. (2012). The Plant-Powered Diet: The Lifelong Eating Plan for Achieving Optimal Health, Beginning Today. New York: The Experiment, LLC.

Plant Stong, Rip Esselstyn. Recipes, Blog, Retreat, and Conference Information: https://plantstrong.com

Prosphoro, additional information on making Greek Holy Bread with printable prayers. https://www.prosphoro.com/aboutprosphorocom

Pukel, S. Holistic Holiday at Sea (Annual Plant-Based Cruise with Classes). Retrieved from https://holisticholidayatsea.com

Pulde, A. M. (2014). Forks Over Knives. Book and video. New York: Simon & Schuster, Inc.

Rouxbe World Class Professional Plant-Based Certification.

Sage Journals, (2013). Consumption of Boiled Greek Coffee is associated with cardiovascular benefits.

Selby, Gaynor, Olive Oil Times, (2015). University of Granada research, Frying in Olive Oil Increases Healthy Phenols.

Veg Rabbis - Jewish Veg, website: https://www.jewishveg.org.

Wolfe, D. (n.d.). BodyMind Institute. Retrieved from David Wolfe Raw Nutrition Certification: https://bodymindinstitute.com/the-exclusive-david-wolfe-nutrition-certification/

Index

A

Air Fried Almonds with Greek Seasoning 130
Air Fried Chickpeas with Greek Seasoning 131
Air Fried Keftedes 76
Almond Coconut Cream 132
Almond Cream Soda 122
Almond Cream Syrup 134
Almond Pate 35
Almond Pulp Cookies 133
Apple Slices with Agave & Cinnamon 95

B

Baklava Nibbles 97
Baklava with Spice Almond Milk Syrup & Dark Chocolate 121
Balsamic Cinnamon Syrup 143
Beer 47
    Beer Battered Blossoms & Veggies 48
    Beer Battered "Cardoona" 49
    Beer Battered Oysters 51
Beer Battered Blossoms & Veggies 48
Beer Batter Recipe 47
Beets 45
    Baby Beets with Cream Cheese & Pistachios 45
    Pickled Beets 94
Bruschetta Greek Style 53

C

Chia Pudding with Whiskey Macerated Raisins 99
Cinnamon Nice Cream 101
Cinnamon Sugar 119
Cracked Marinated Olives 54

D

Dark Chocolate Dipped Figs with Pistachios & Anise Dust 107
Dedication 3
Definitions 10
    Mezethakia 10
    Plant-Based Diet 10
Dips & Smears 34
    Almond Pate 35
    Beetroot Hummus 37
    Cilantro Hummus 37
    Greek Roasted Eggplant Spread 39
    How to Roast Beet(s) 37
    Hummus 35
    Raw Zucchini Hummus 40
    Roasted Red Bell Pepper Hummus 40
    Santorini Yellow Fava Hummus 41
    Walnut Spread 43
Dukkah with Hemp 135

F

Feta Plate 60
Fig & Anise Energy Bites 103
Fig Fruit & Nut Salami 108
Fig Granita 105
Fig & Raisin Fruit Paste with Anise & Cinnamon 141
Figs 93
    Dark Chocolate Dipped Figs with Pistachios & Anise Dust 107
    Fig & Anise
    Energy Bites 103
    Fig Fruit & Nut Salami 108
    Fig Granita 105
    Sweet Spiced Pickled Figs Stuffed with Feta 93
Fried Polenta 63
Fruit Plate 66
Fruit with Almond Cream Syrup & Yogurt 109

G

Gazpacho 61
Greek Coffee 123
Greek Coffee Glaze 118
Greek Gazpacho 61
Greek Guac 65
Greek Herbs List 152
Greek Kale Chips 139
Greek Nachos 75
Greek Oyster Po Boy 51
Greek Roasted Eggplant Spread 39
Greek Seasoning Blend 142
Greek Spice List 151
Greek Whipped Coffee Frappe 124
Green Falafels 58
Green Gyro 73
Gremolata 142
Grilled Greek Toasts 143
Grilled Pita Breads 143
Grilled Veggie Platter 71
Gyro with Grilled Veggies Slider 70

H

Horta - Greens 79
Horta Hand Pie 79
How to Cook Lentils 77
How to Roast Beet(s) 37
Hummus 35
    Beetroot Hummus 37
    Cilantro Hummus 37
    Plain Hummus 35
    Raw Zucchini Hummus 40
    Roasted Red Bell Pepper Hummus 40
    Santorini Yellow Fava Hummus 41

I

Iced Orange Tea with Cinnamon & Mint 126
Introduction 8

K

Kale 139
  Dehydrated Kale Chips 139
  Greek Kale Chips 139
  Oven Baked Kale Chips 139
Keftedes 76
  Air Fried Keftedes 76
  How to Cook Lentils 77
  Shallow Fry keftedes on Stove-top 76
Koliva 78

L

Lemony Greek Roasted Potatoes 80
Loukoumades with Flax Seeds & Greek Coffee Glaze 118

M

Medjool Dates with Walnut Stuffing 110
Mint & Cinnamon Simple Syrup 143
More Stuff
  Air Fried Almonds with Greek Seasoning 130
  Air Fried Chickpeas with Greek Seasoning 131
  Almond Coconut Cream 132
  Almond Cream Syrup 134
  Balsamic Cinnamon Syrup 143
  Dukkah with Hemp 135
  Fig & Raisin Fruit Paste with Anise & Cinnamon 141
  Greek Kale Chips 139
  Greek Seasoning Blend 142
  Gremolata 142
  Grilled Pita Breads 143
  Mint & Cinnamon Simple Syrup 143
  Pita Chips 145
  Prosforo - Greek Offering Bread 146
  Schug 148
  Zaatar Crackers 150

N

Naked Baklava 111
Naked Fig & Nut Cookie - Skaltsounia 112
Noshes & Nibbles 44
  Air Fried Keftedes 76
  Baby Beets with Cream Cheese & Pistachios 45
  Beer Battered Blossoms & Veggies 48
  Beer Battered "Cardoona" 49
  Beer Battered Oysters 51
  Beer Batter Recipe 47
  Bruschetta Greek Style 53
  Cardoona 49
  Feta Plate 60
  Fried Polenta 63
  Fruit Plate 66
  Greek Gazpacho 61
  Greek Guac 65
  Greek Nachos 75
  Greek Oyster Po Boy 51
  Green Falafels 58
  Green Gyro 73
  Grilled Veggie Platter 71
  Gyro with Grilled Veggies Slider 70
  Horta - Greens 79
  Horta Hand Pie 79
  Olive Tapenade 55
  Persian Pizza 81
  Power Greens in Phyllo 83
  Stuffed Celery & Other Veggies 85
  Tomato Keftedes 84
  Veggie Platter 69
  White Beans on Grilled Greek Toast 86

O

Olive Tapenade 55
Orange Spiced Wine Syrup 144

P

Pantry 151
  Greek Herbs List 152
  Greek-ish Pantry 151
  Greek Spice List 151
Persian Pizza 81
Pickled Beets 94
Pickled Carrots 90
Pickled Grapes 89
Pickled Prunes 90
Pickled Red Onions 89
Pickled Turnips 91
Pita Chips 145
Pita Cinnamon Toast 119
Polenta 63
Potatoes 13
  Greek Potato Salad 13
  Lemony Greek Roasted Potatoes 80
  Potato Salad with Mint Dressing 16
  Potato Skins Greek Style with Lemon & Oregano 74
Power Greens in Phyllo 83
Prosforo - Greek Offering Bread 146

Q

Quick Pickles 93
  Pickled Beets 94
  Pickled Carrots 90
  Pickled Grapes 89
  Pickled Prunes 90
  Pickled Red Onions 89
  Pickled Turnips 91

R

References 155
Roasted Fruit with Balsamic Cinnamon Syrup 113
Roasted Pumpkin Spoon Sweet 117

S

Salad Dressings
  Greek Hemp Dressing 31
  Greek Salad Dressing 31
  Hummus Salad Dressing 31
  Mint Salad Dressing 32
  Salad with Greek Hemp Dressing Photo 31
  Tahini Dressing 33
  Tzatziki Dressing 33

Salads 11
  Chopped Salad with Chickpeas 17
  Creamy Cucumber & Tomato Salad with Tzatziki Dressing 19
  Fattoush Salad 23
  Fruit Salad with Mint & Cinnamon Simple Syrup 27
  Greek Potato Salad 13
  Greek Salad 12
  Greek Village Salad 19
  Greek Village Salad with Tzatziki 19
  Holiday Tabouli 25
  Lentil Salad 21
  Massaged Kale Salad with Hummus Dressing 15
  Orange Slices & Pomegranate Seeds in Spiced Wine Syrup 29
  Potato Salad with Mint Dressing 16
  Tabouli with Celery & Mint 25
  Tomatoes with Fresh Mint 26

Schug 148
Shepherd's Tea or Mountain Tea 127
Shopping List 153
Sips & Swigs 125
  Almond Cream Soda 122
  Greek Coffee 123
  Greek Whipped Coffee Frappe 124
  Iced Orange Tea with Cinnamon & Mint 126
  Shepherd's Tea or Mountain Tea 127
  Sparkling Mint Punch with Wheatgrass 128

Sparkling Mint Punch with Wheatgrass 128
Spiced Almond Milk Syrup 121
Spoon Sweets 115
Stuffed Celery & Other Veggies 85
Sweets
  Almond Pulp Cookies 133
  Apple Slices with Agave & Cinnamon 95
  Baklava with Spice Almond Milk Syrup & Dark Chocolate 121
  Chia Pudding with Whiskey Macerated Raisins 99
  Cinnamon Nice Cream with Baklava Spiced Nuts 101
  Cinnamon Sugar 119
  Dark Chocolate Dipped Figs with Pistachios & Anise Dust 107
  Fig & Anise Energy Bites 103
  Fig Fruit & Nut Salami 108
  Fig Granita 105
  Fruit with Almond Cream Syrup & Yogurt 109
  Greek Coffee Glaze 118
  Greek Coffee Granita with Cardamom 102
  Loukoumades with Flax Seeds & Greek Coffee Glaze 118
  Medjool Dates with Walnut Stuffing 110
  Naked Baklava 111
  Naked Fig & Nut Cookie - Skaltsounia 112
  Pita Cinnamon Toast 119
  Roasted Fruit with Balsamic Cinnamon Syrup 113
  Roasted Pumpkin Spoon Sweet 117
  Spiced Almond Milk Syrup 121
  Spoon Sweets 115

Sweet Spiced Pickled Figs Stuffed with Feta 93

T

Tomatoes with Fresh Mint 26
Tomato Fritters 57
Tomato Keftedes 84

V

Veggie Fritters 57
  Spinach Fritters 57
  Tomato Fritters 57
  Zucchini Fritters 57
Veggie Platter 69

W

Walnut Spread 43
Wet Walnuts in Spiced Wine Syrup 144
White Beans on Grilled Greek Toast 86

Z

Zaatar Crackers 150

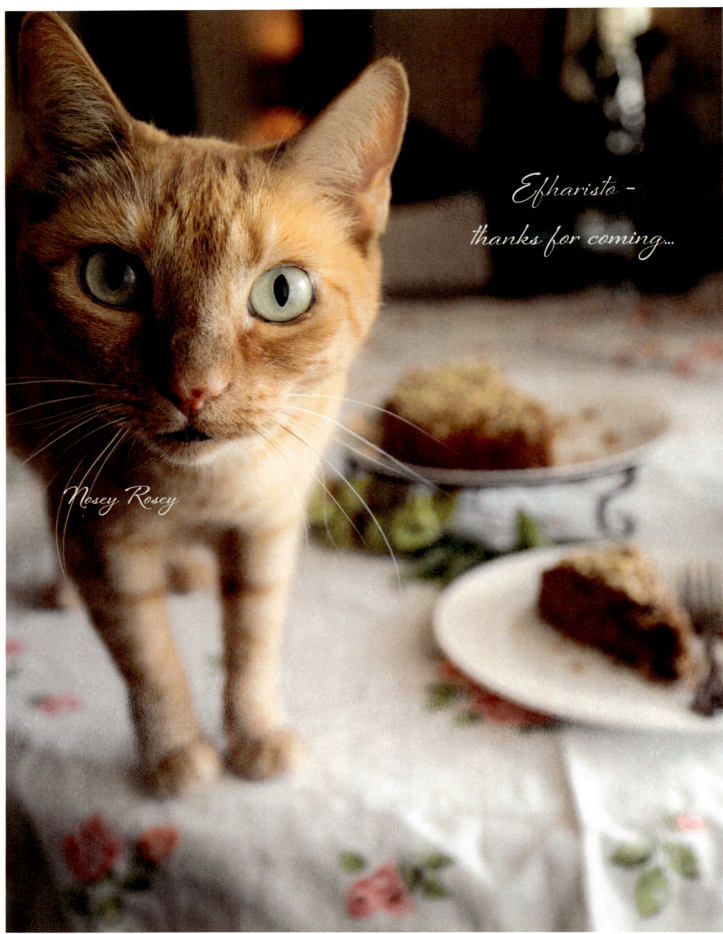

Na eisai kala!

I wish you well -

peace & blessings on you & yours

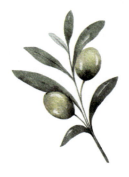

Made in the USA
Las Vegas, NV
07 October 2023

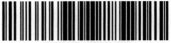

78723770R00098